PULMONARY
FUNCTION
TESTING

REUBEN M. CHERNIACK, M.D.

Professor and Chairman
Department of Medicine
The University of Manitoba
Faculty of Medicine
Winnipeg, Canada

W. B. SAUNDERS COMPANY
Philadelphia • London • Toronto

W. B. Saunders Company: West Washington Square
Philadelphia, Pa. 19105

1 St. Anne's Road
Eastbourne, East Sussex BN21 3UN, England

1 Goldthorne Avenue
Toronto, Ontario M8Z 5T9, Canada

Library of Congress Cataloging in Publication Data

Cherniack, Reuben M

Pulmonary function testing.

Includes index.

1. Pulmonary function tests.   2. Respiration.   I. Title
  [DNLM: 1. Respiratory function tests. WB284 C521p]

RC734.P84C48   616.2′4′0754   77–75533

ISBN 0–7216–2528–2

Pulmonary Muscle Testing   ISBN 0-7216-2528-2

Last digit is the print number: 9   8   7   6   5   4   3

PREFACE

In recent years the knowledge of the physiologic disturbances present in patients suffering from respiratory diseases has increased considerably, and there has been an explosion of new tests of pulmonary function. An increased awareness of the importance of even simple tests of pulmonary function has led to the development of pulmonary function laboratories in most hospitals. Most physicians now recognize that the measurement of the amount of disability present is an essential component of the clinical assessment in any patient who complains of respiratory symptoms. What is not yet accepted is the fact that this does not necessitate referral to a pulmonary function laboratory. Valuable information can be obtained in the office or at the bedside by analysis of the forced expiratory volume, which can be estimated with a simple spirometer while examining the patient. In addition, much can be learned by noting the onset of breathlessness and tachycardia when the patient engages in a form of activity to which he is accustomed, such as climbing a flight of stairs or walking. But these simple assessments yield information that is insufficient in many clinical situations, and more specific laboratory studies of pulmonary function are necessary.

The degree of sophistication and complexity of the pulmonary function tests that are used varies widely, depending on local circumstances. In addition to the simple ventilatory function studies, measurements of the mechanical properties of the lung can be of considerable value, and in patients who are critically ill or suffer from chronic illness, gas exchange and acid-base status are essential.

Used judiciously, the assessment of pulmonary function enables the physician to recognize early disease, to follow its progress, and to prescribe proper therapy directed at improving the disturbances in pulmonary function. When surgery (particularly the removal of lung tissue) is contemplated, the patient's ability to tolerate an anesthetic or narcotic or the removal of lung tissue can be assessed, and this information may be used as a guide to the preparation and postoperative care of the patient.

Many allied health professionals are being asked to perform and interpret most of these tests of pulmonary function without sufficient background training and knowledge. The purpose of this text is to present the background information necessary to understand normal pulmonary function and the disturbances that occur in disease. On this foundation the basis of the various tests that are used to determine pulmonary function and to assess disability are discussed, along with their interpretation. In order to determine how well these principles are understood by the reader, the opportunity for self-assessment with multiple choice questions and case examples is provided.

Acknowledgment

I am grateful to Laurayne Rusak for her extensive efforts in typing the manuscript and proofreading, and to Kathy Kork for the diagrams.

Reuben M. Cherniack

CONTENTS

Section I

BASIC CONSIDERATIONS

INTRODUCTION

To those who are not pulmonary physiologists, the vast number of terms, symbols, and abbreviations used in discussing pulmonary physiology or tests of function are often confusing. But in fact there is some logic in the symbols that are used as abbreviations and, once understood, there is usually no difficulty in following any discussion or publication dealing with pulmonary function. Therefore the first chapter of this book is devoted to a summary of the basic terminology you will be expected to know.

In the next few chapters we will deal with the way in which air and blood are transported into the lungs, gas exchange across the alveolocapillary membrane, the transport of oxygen and carbon dioxide in the blood, and the impact of the respiratory system on acid-base balance in the body.

Contraction of the respiratory muscles during inspiration brings fresh ambient air into lungs. The ambient air, whose total pressure is 760 torr at sea level, contains 20.94 per cent oxygen, 0.04 per cent carbon dioxide, and 79 per cent nitrogen, with partial pressures of 159, 0.3, and 600 torr respectively.

The total pressure of the gases in the lung is also equal to the ambient barometric pressure. However, when the air enters the lungs it becomes diluted by and saturated with water vapor that evaporates from the surface of the tracheobronchial tree. Water vapor, like other gases, exerts a partial pressure, but unlike other gases, its partial pressure depends almost entirely on the temperature and is virtually unaffected by the barometric pressure. At normal body temperature (37°C) the partial pressure of water vapor is 47 torr. In the alveoli the gas is further diluted by the presence of carbon dioxide that has passed from blood in the pulmonary capillaries into the alveoli. In the alveolar air there is approximately 15 per cent oxygen, 6 per cent carbon dioxide, and 79 per cent nitrogen.

Because of the presence of water vapor, the pressure of dry alveolar gas will be 47 torr less than the barometric pressure. This is important, because analysis of the gases present in alveolar air or expired air is reported in terms of the dry gas. To calculate the partial pressure of a particular gas in the alveolar or expired gas, its fractional concentration is multiplied by the barometric pressure minus the water vapor pressure.

Thus $P_A = F_A \times$ (barometric pressure -47)

or

$P_E = F_E \times$ (barometric pressure -47)

where P represents the partial pressure and F the fractional concentration of a gas in the alveolar air (A) or the expired air (E). In healthy lungs the partial pressures of oxygen, carbon dioxide, and nitrogen in the alveolar air are approximately 100, 40, and 570 torr.

The blood that enters the pulmonary capillaries has come from the tissues and therefore has a low oxygen content (P_{O_2} about 40 torr) and high carbon dioxide content (P_{CO_2} about 46 torr). Because the partial pressures of the gases in the alveolar air and the capillary blood are different, oxygen diffuses from the alveoli into the capillary blood and carbon dioxide diffuses into the alveoli. The oxygen-depleted and carbon-dioxide-enriched alveolar gas leaves through the airway during the ensuing expiration, while the blood that has taken up oxygen and given off carbon dioxide enters the systemic arteries and travels to the tissues. Here oxygen diffuses into the cells, and the carbon dioxide that has been produced in the cells is taken up by the blood. This venous blood, in turn, is once again transported to the lungs and there it exchanges gases with the alveolar gas.

Chapter 1

ABBREVIATIONS AND DEFINITIONS

ABBREVIATIONS

Many of the abbreviations used in pulmonary physiology consist of a series of primary symbols that relate to a

5

primary variable, such as a physical quantity (volume or pressure) or a calculated parameter. These primary symbols may be modified by superscripts that denote a time derivative or mean value, and are often qualified by secondary symbols noted as subscripts that specify the anatomic location or physiologic derivation of the measurement. They, in turn, may be followed by further symbols to indicate molecular species, and these symbols are separated from the main term by a comma.

PRIMARY SYMBOLS

Gas Exchange

C   Concentration in blood phase
D   Diffusing capacity
F   Fractional concentration of a gas
P   Pressure, gas or blood
Q   Volume of blood
R   Respiratory exchange ratio
S   Saturation of Hb in the blood phase
V   Gas volume

Pulmonary Mechanics

C   Compliance
f   Respiratory frequency
G   Conductance
R   Resistance

SUPERSCRIPTS

A dot above the symbol denotes a time derivative such as $\dot{V}$–volume per unit time (i.e., ventilation in

liters per minute) or $\dot{Q}$ (blood flow per minute).
A line above the symbol denotes a mean value such as
$\bar{v}$ — mixed venous.

SECONDARY SYMBOLS OR SUBSCRIPTS

Anatomic Location

aw	Airway
bs	Body surface
cw	Chest wall
es	Esophageal
L	Lung (pulmonary)
LA	Left atrium
LV	Left ventricle
PA	Pulmonary artery
pl	Pleural

Gases

Ar	Argon
CO	Carbon monoxide
CO$_2$	Carbon dioxide
N$_2$	Nitrogen
O$_2$	Oxygen
SF$_6$	Sulfur hexafluoride
Xe	Xenon

Gas Phase

A	Alveolar gas
B	Barometric
D	Dead space or wasted gas

E	Expired gas
ET	End tidal gas
I	Inspired gas
T	Tidal gas
TG	Thoracic gas

Blood Phase

a	Arterial blood
b	Blood in general
c	Capillary blood
ċ	Pulmonary end-capillary blood
s	Shunt
t	Total
v	Venous blood
v̄	Mixed venous blood

Pulmonary Mechanics

ds	Downstream
dyn	Dynamic
el	Elastic
max	Maximal
st	Static
us	Upstream

CONDITIONS

ATPD	Ambient temperature and pressure, dry
ATPS	Saturated with water vapor at ambient temperature and pressure
BTPS	Body conditions: saturated with water vapor at body temperature and ambient pressure

STPD Standard conditions: temperature 0 °C, pressure 760 mm Hg (torr)

DEFINITIONS

Abbreviations are also used for almost all parameters of lung function. The following lists most of these abbreviations and their definition.

LUNG VOLUME COMPARTMENTS

CC Closing capacity
The volume of gas left in the lungs when the rapid change in "marker" gas concentration occurs (this is thought to be the volume at which airway closure begins) from an alveolar plateau during a slow expiratory vital capacity maneuver.

Thus $$CC = CV + RV$$

CV Closing volume
The volume of gas exhaled after there has been a rapid change in the concentration of an inert "marker" gas from an alveolar plateau during a slow expiratory vital capacity maneuver.

ERV Expiratory reserve volume
The maximum volume of air that can be exhaled from the end-expiratory level, or from functional residual capacity (FRC).

FRC Functional residual capacity
The volume of air remaining in the lungs at the end of an

ordinary expiration (i.e., at the resting level or end-expiratory level).

IC   Inspiratory capacity
The maximal volume of air that can be inhaled, i.e., to total lung capacity (TLC) from the end-expiratory level i.e., from functional residual capacity (FRC).

IRV   Inspiratory reserve volume
The maximal volume of air that can be inhaled, i.e., to total lung capacity (TLC) over and above the tidal volume.

RV   Residual volume
The volume of air remaining in the lungs after a maximal expiration.

Thus $$RV = TLC - VC$$

TLC   Total lung capacity
The sum of all the compartments of the lung, or the volume of air in the lungs at maximum inspiration.

VC   Vital capacity
The maximum volume of air that can be expelled after a maximum inspiration, i.e., from total lung capacity (TLC).

V_T Tidal volume
The volume of air inhaled or exhaled with each breath during breathing.

SPIROMETRY

$FEV_{1.0}$ Forced expiratory volume in one second
The volume of air expelled in one second during a forced

expiration, starting at full inspiration, i.e., at total lung capacity (TLC).

FVC   Forced vital capacity
The volume of air expired during a rapid forced expiration starting at full inspiration, i.e., at total lung capacity (TLC) and ending at residual volume.

MEFV   Maximum expiratory flow-volume curves
The plotted relationship between flow and volume during a forced vital capacity maneuver.

MMF   Maximum mid-expiratory flow rate
The mean rate of expiratory air flow between 25 and 75 per cent of the forced expiratory vital capacity.

PEF   Peak expiratory flow
The greatest flow that can be obtained during a forced expiration starting from full inflation of the lung, i.e., at total lung capacity (TLC).

$\dot{V}_{max}$ Maximum flow
This is usually expressed at a particular lung volume. Flow rates at 50 per cent and 25 per cent of vital capacity are often used.

AIR FLOW RESISTANCE

EPP   Equal pressure point
The point in the airways at which the pressure in the airways is equal to the pressure surrounding it during a forced expiration.

G_{aw} Airways conductance

The reciprocal of resistance, i.e., the airflow (in liters per second) achieved by a 1 cm H_2O pressure difference between the alveoli and mouth, and expressed in ℓ/sec/cm H_2O.

G_{aw}/V_L Specific conductance
The value of conductance is corrected for the lung volume at which the measurement was made and expressed in units/sec/cm H_2O.

R_{aw} Airways resistance
The pressure difference between the alveoli and the mouth required to produce an air flow of 1 liter per second. It is expressed in cm H_2O/ℓ/sec.

R_{ds} Downstream resistance
The pressure difference between the equal pressure point (EPP) and the mouth required to produce a $\dot{V}_{max}$ of 1 liter per second. It is expressed in cm H_2O/ℓ/sec.

R_L Total pulmonary resistance
The ratio of the pressure difference required to produce flow between the pleural surface and the mouth and flow at the mouth. It is expressed in cm H_2O/ℓ/sec.

R_{us} Upstream resistance
The pressure difference between the alveoli and the equal pressure point (EPP) required to produce a $\dot{V}_{max}$ of 1 liter per second. It is expressed in cm H_2O/ℓ/sec.

ELASTIC RESISTANCE

C Compliance
A measure of distensibility—the volume change produced by a unit of pressure.

C_{cw} Chest wall compliance
The change in lung volume produced by an increase in
pressure across the chest wall, i.e., the difference in pressure between the pleural surface and the outside of the
chest.

C_{dyn} Dynamic compliance
The lung compliance during breathing, i.e., the ratio of
the tidal volume to the change in trans-pulmonary pressure from end-expiration to end-inspiration.

C_L Lung compliance
The volume change produced by an increase in a unit
change in pressure across the lung, i.e., between the
pleural surface and the mouth. It is expressed in ℓ/cm
H_2O.

C_{st} Static compliance
The compliance determined between points where airflow is obstructed for a second or more. The trans-
pulmonary pressure is related to the absolute lung
volume over the entire range of lung volume from total
lung capacity (TLC) to residual volume (RV).

C/V_L Specific compliance
The lung compliance is corrected for the lung volume at
which the measurement was made, and is expressed in
units/ℓ.

E Elastance
The trans-pulmonary pressure difference divided by the
volume change, i.e., pressure per unit of volume change.

P_{st} Static pressure
Static trans-pulmonary pressure at a specified lung volume.

INTERACTION OF ELASTIC AND FLOW RESISTANCE

MBC or MVV   Maximum voluntary ventilation
The maximum volume of air that can be breathed in 12 to 15 seconds. It is expressed in ℓ/min.

RC   Time constant
An electrical analogue of impedances in the lung—the product of resistance and compliance.

W   Mechanical work of breathing.

VENTILATION AND PERFUSION

$C(a\text{-}v)_{O_2}$ Arteriovenous oxygen content difference
The difference in oxygen concentration between the arterial and the venous blood.

Dead-space-like ventilation
Ventilation of poorly perfused or non-perfused alveoli, i.e., high ventilation/perfusion ratio.

Index of intrapulmonary mixing
The concentration of nitrogen in the alveolar gas after breathing 100 per cent oxygen for 7 minutes.

Mixing efficiency
The ratio of the theoretical over the actual number of breaths taken to reach 90 per cent equilibrium for helium between the lungs and the spirometer in a closed circuit.

$P_{A_{O_2}}$ Alveolar P_{O_2}

The ideal partial pressure of oxygen in the alveoli, which is estimated from the inspired oxygen, the $P_{a_{CO_2}}$ and the respiratory exchange ratio (R) by the alveolar air equation. A simplified version of the alveolar air equation is

$$P_{A_{O_2}} = P_{I_{O_2}} - \frac{P_{a_{CO_2}}}{R}$$

$P(A\text{-}a)_{O_2}$ Alveolar-arterial P_{O_2} difference or gradient

An overall measure of the efficiency of the lung as a gas exchanger. In a perfect ventilation/perfusion system, $P_{A_{O_2}}$ is equal to $P_{a_{O_2}}$. In healthy subjects, the A-a gradient is 5 to 15 mm Hg (torr).

$\dot{V}_A$ Alveolar ventilation

That part of the total ventilation ($\dot{V}_E$) that takes part in gas exchange.

V_D Dead space or physiologic dead space

That part of the tidal breath (V_T) that does not take part in gas exchange.

$\dot{V}_E$ Minute ventilation

The amount of air breathed per minute.

Venous admixture

Shunting of venous blood into arterialized blood.

Venous-admixture-like perfusion

Perfusion of poorly ventilated or non-ventilated alveoli, i.e., low ventilation/perfusion ratio.

GAS TRANSFER

CO   Extraction
The proportion of the inspired volume of carbon monoxide that is transferred across the alveolocapillary membrane.

$\mathbf{D}_{L_{CO}}$ Diffusing capacity for carbon monoxide
The ability of the lungs to transfer carbon monoxide from the alveolar air into pulmonary capillary blood. It is expressed as ml/min/mm Hg.

BLOOD GAS STATUS

Hypercapnia or Hypercarbia
A greater than normal arterial carbon dioxide tension.

Hyperoxia
A greater than normal amount of oxygen in the air, blood, or tissues.

Hypocapnia or Hypocarbia
A lower than normal arterial carbon dioxide tension.

Hypoxemia
A lower than normal partial pressure of oxygen, or oxygen saturation of hemoglobin, or both.

Hypoxia
A lower than normal amount of oxygen in the air, blood, or tissues.

Normocapnia or Normocarbia
A normal arterial carbon dioxide tension.

Normoxia
A normal amount of oxygen in the air, blood, or tissues.

Torr
The pressure required to support a column of mercury 1 mm high. Synonymous with partial pressure, or mm Hg.

ACID-BASE STATUS

Acid
A substance that can donate hydrogen ions (H^+).

$$e.g., HCL \longrightarrow H^+ + Cl^+$$

Acidemia
A state of the systemic arterial plasma in which the pH is significantly less than 7.35.

Acidosis
The result of any process which, by itself, adds excess carbon dioxide (respiratory acidosis) or nonvolatile acids (metabolic acidosis) to the arterial blood.

Alkalemia
A state of the systemic arterial plasma in which the pH is significantly greater than 7.45.

Alkalosis
The result of any process that, by itself, diminishes acids (respiratory alkalosis) or increases bases (metabolic alkalosis) in the arterial blood.

Anion
A negatively charged ion that migrates toward an anode.

Base
A substance that can accept hydrogen ions.

Buffer
A substance that interacts with acids or bases to minimize changes in pH.

Cation
A positively charged ion that migrates toward a cathode.

Chemical equilibrium
A situation that exists when the rate of a reaction in one direction is equal to the rate in the opposite direction. This does not mean that the constituents on both sides of the reaction are equal.

pH
The negative logarithm, to the base 10, of the concentration of free hydrogen ions in a solution.

EXERCISE

Maximal $\dot{V}_{O_2}$ Maximal oxygen intake
The maximum oxygen consumption attainable during exercise, usually expressed as Max $\dot{V}_{O_2}$/kg of body weight. This may be measured directly, but is usually extrapolated from the $\dot{V}_{O_2}$ and cardiac frequency.

METS
The oxygen consumption during exercise, expressed as a multiple of the resting oxygen consumption.

Chapter 2

PULMONARY MECHANICS

In order to expand the chest during inspiration, the respiratory muscles must develop sufficient force to overcome the resistances offered by the respiratory apparatus and the gas in the respiratory tract. The respiratory apparatus is composed of the lungs and the chest wall (i.e., the chest cage, the diaphragm, and the

19

abdominal contents), each of which has an elastic force, and the tracheobronchial tree, which offers resistance to airflow.

ELASTIC FORCES

When all the respiratory muscles are relaxed and there is no air moving in or out of the lungs (as is the situation at the end of a normal expiration), there is still a volume of air in the lungs. This volume of gas in the lungs is called the **functional residual capacity** (FRC), and is determined by the balance of the elastic forces exerted by the lungs and chest wall. Although this position of the chest is often referred to as the resting level, neither the lungs nor the chest wall are at their resting position. The elastic recoil of the lungs is actually pulling in an expiratory direction, and this is being prevented by the elastic force of the chest wall, which is pulling outwards with an equal pressure. This is illustrated in Figure 2–1, in which a model of the lung-chest wall system in the form of a two plate piston within a container is depicted. Note that each of the plates is attached to a set of springs, that the two sets of springs are pulling in opposite directions, and that a rubber balloon representing the pleural cavity separates the two plates. The springs attached to the left plate represent the elastic resistance of the lung, and those attached to the right plate represent that of the chest wall. In this particular situation the piston is stationary and at its "resting position" because the forces that are being exerted by the two sets of springs are equal. Clearly this is analogous to the equilibrium situation that exists in the human thorax at the resting level or functional residual capacity.

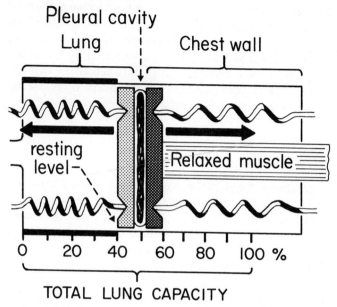

Figure 2–1. The elastic forces of the lungs and the chest wall at the "resting level" in a mechanical analogue. The springs on the left represent the force of lung elasticity, and those on the right represent the elastic forces of the chest wall. The forces being exerted by the two springs are equal, so the piston is stationary. This is analogous to the situation in the human at functional residual capacity.

The maximum excursions of the respiratory apparatus in both the inspiratory and expiratory directions are also determined by a balance of forces — the elastic characteristics of the respiratory apparatus and the muscle forces that are applied to the apparatus. Thus when the lungs are inflated maximally, the elastic forces of the respiratory system are balanced by the maximum inspiratory muscle forces. Similarly, there is a limit to the amount of air that can be expelled from the lungs and, after a maximal expiration, the elastic forces (mainly the chest wall) tending to expand the lungs are balanced by the maximum expiratory muscle forces. Between these two extremes, the relationship between the elastic forces of the lung and the chest wall is related to the lung volume.

LUNG VOLUME

Breathing takes place within the framework of the boundaries of the maximum excursions of the respiratory apparatus. The maximum volume of air that can be contained in the lung is called the **total lung capacity** (TLC), which is often considered to consist of several subdivisions or compartments. Figure 2–2 indicates the subdivisions as proportions of the total lung capacity be-

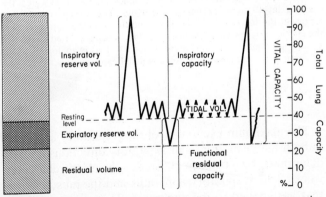

Figure 2–2. The subdivisions of lung volume shown as a proportion of total lung capacity. The block diagram on the left is included for future reference in other figures.

cause, although their absolute values vary considerably even in healthy persons (depending on the age, sex, and size of the person), the proportion of the total lung capacity that each of the components occupies is remarkably similar.

As has already been pointed out, the quantity of air remaining in the lungs at the end of a normal expiration is called the **functional residual capacity** (FRC). The FRC is normally about 40 per cent of the TLC and is made up of two components — the **expiratory reserve volume** (ERV), which is the maximum volume of air that can be expired beyond the FRC (about 15 per cent of TLC), and the **residual volume** (RV), which is the amount of air left in the lungs at the end of this maximal expiration (about 25 per cent of TLC).

The **inspiratory capacity** (IC), which is the maximum volume of air that can be inspired from the FRC, normally averages about 60 per cent of the TLC. Clearly the **tidal volume** (V_T) is a component of this subdivision. The **inspiratory reserve volume** (IRV) is the maximal volume of air that can be inspired, over and above the tidal volume, from the FRC.

The **vital capacity** (VC), is the maximal amount of air that a subject is able to expire after a maximal inspiration (or inspire after a maximal expiration). Clearly the VC, which is normally about 75 per cent of the TLC, may also be considered the sum of several compartments (e.g., IC + ERV).

ELASTIC FORCES AND LUNG VOLUME

In Figure 2–3 the mechanical analogue is utilized to illustrate the relationship between the elastic forces of the lung and chest wall at different lung volumes. When the piston is pulled out as far as possible, a situation analogous to that which exists at TLC, the springs representing the elastic forces of the lung are stretched, while those representing the elastic forces of the chest wall are compressed and actually attempting to re-expand (Fig. 2–3A). At TLC, then, both the elastic forces are exerted in an expiratory direction so that the piston (or the lung) has a propensity to recoil toward a smaller volume.

As the piston is allowed to return toward its original position, the stretch on both springs diminishes. At a particular point (about 67 per cent of TLC), the "chest wall" spring is completely relaxed and is not exerting a force in any direction, while the "lung" spring continues to exert a force in an expiratory direction (Fig. 2–3B). Thus the piston (and the lungs) tend to move in an expiratory direction until the pull of the "chest wall" spring becomes equal to that of the lung.

If the piston is pushed past its resting position, as would occur if one were to expire to a volume less than FRC, there is less stretch of the "lung" spring so that its

Figure 2–3. The elastic forces of the lung and the chest wall at maximum inspiration (TLC), at approximately 67 per cent of the total lung capacity, and at maximum expiration (RV). On the left the stretch on the springs of the mechanical analogue is shown. In the center the relative propensity of the forces of the lung and chest wall are depicted, and on the right the lung volume at which these forces are acting is represented.

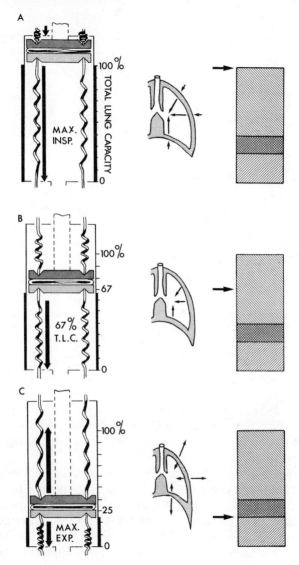

Figure 2–3. *See legend on the opposite page.*

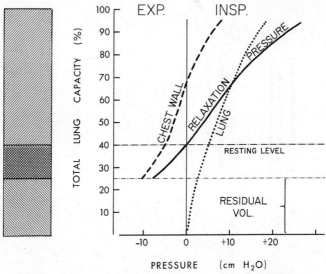

Figure 2–4. Depicted is the pressure derived at different lung volumes when a subject relaxes against a complete obstruction (relaxation pressure). This pressure is the resultant net balance between the elastic forces of the lung and the chest wall at all levels of lung volume.

retractile force is small, while the "chest wall" spring is stretched more, so that its tendency to recoil increases (Fig. 2–3*C*). In this situation the net force is in an inspiratory direction, so there will be a propensity for the volume to increase until the pull of the two sets of springs in opposite directions is equal.

A plot of the relationship between the elastic forces of the lungs and chest wall at different lung volumes in the human is illustrated in Figure 2–4. Also shown is the resultant net balance between these two forces (termed **relaxation pressure**), which is derived by having the subject relax against a complete obstruction at different lung volumes. In this figure pressures tending to increase lung volume are negative and those tending to decrease lung volume are positive. As in the model, the forces exerted by the lung and chest wall are equal and pulling in opposite directions at FRC, so the relaxation pressure is zero, or atmospheric. When the lung is inflated above FRC, the force of the lung tending to empty it is greater than that of the chest wall tending to fill it, and the relaxation pressure is positive. It becomes even more positive at very high lung volumes, when the lung and chest wall forces both act in an expiratory direction. At lung volumes below FRC, the pull of the chest wall in an inspiratory direction is greater than the pull of the lungs in an expiratory direction, so the relaxation pressure is negative. As was seen in the mechanical analogue, there is a propensity for the lung volume to return to the "resting level" at lung volumes higher or lower than FRC.

COMPLIANCE

The elastic resistance or distensibility of the springs we have used in the mechanical analogue can be described by the force necessary to stretch and hold them at a certain length. The distensibility of the respiratory apparatus can also be described by its force-displacement characteristics. Distensibility can be determined by either altering the pressure and noting the volume change that results, or by changing the volume and noting the pressure required to maintain the new volume.

The pressure-volume characteristics of the respiratory apparatus (or of the chest wall or the lungs) are usually expressed in terms of the **compliance,** which is the change in volume per unit change in pressure across each part of the system.

$$\text{Compliance} = \frac{\text{change in volume } (\Delta V)}{\text{change in pressure } (\Delta P)}$$

Thus the compliance of the respiratory apparatus is $\Delta V/\Delta P_{chest}$; the compliance of the lungs is $\Delta V/\Delta P_{lung}$; and the compliance of the chest wall is $\Delta V/\Delta P_{wall}$.

The distensibility can also be expressed as the change in pressure per unit of volume change, in which case it is called the **elastic resistance** or **elastance**; the values obtained are clearly the reciprocal of the compliance.

When a spring (or lung) is easy to distend (elastic resistance is low), it has a high compliance. If it is difficult to distend (elastic resistance is high), it has a low compliance. An example of the elastic behavior (or compliance) of three different springs (or lungs) is shown in Figure 2–5. The application of a pressure of 5 cm H_2O to healthy lungs results in an "inspiration" of 1 liter of air, so that their compliance is 1.0/5 or 0.20 ℓ/cm H_2O (Fig. 2–5A). Figure 2–5B illustrates that the application of a pressure of 5 cm H_2O to lungs that have lost elasticity (as in emphysema) results in an "inspiration" of 2 liters of air; in other words, the compliance is increased to 2.0/5 or 0.40 ℓ/cm H_2O. When the lungs are stiff (as in pulmonary fibrosis) the same pressure change results in a volume change of only 0.5 liter and the compliance is reduced to 0.5/5 or 0.10 ℓ/cm H_2O (Fig. 2–5C).

Figure 2–5. The stretch on the springs represents the distention of the lungs produced by a change in applied or distending pressure of 5 cm H_2O in normal lungs (A), lungs that have lost elasticity (B), and lungs that are fibrotic (C). The change in volume induced by the change in pressure is also plotted.

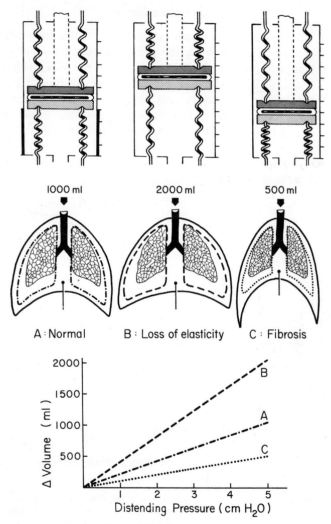

A : Normal   B : Loss of elasticity   C : Fibrosis

Figure 2–5. *See legend on the opposite page.*

Static Compliance

In practice, the elastic properties of the lung are assessed by determining the static elastic component of the applied pressure (usually esophageal pressure, which is a useful approximation of pleural pressure) over the range of the inspiratory and expiratory vital capacity. This is then plotted as a static pressure-volume curve of the lung (Fig. 2–6). It should be apparent that this is the same as the curve depicting lung recoil in Figure 2–4. An example of the static pressure volume curve found when there is a loss of lung elastic recoil, as in emphy-

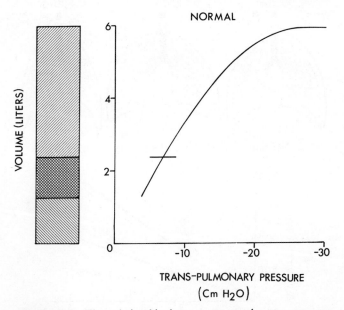

Figure 2–6. The relationship between trans-pulmonary pressure and lung volume (static pressure volume curve of the lung) in a healthy individual is shown. As is seen on the lung volume graph, the horizontal line on the pressure curve represents the resting level or functional residual capacity.

sema, is shown in Figure 2–7, and when there is an increase in lung elastic recoil, as in lung fibrosis, is shown in Figure 2–8. As can be seen, the curve is shifted upward (lung volume is greater) and to the left (pressure is lower) in the patient with emphysema, and down (lung volume is less) and to the right (pressure is greater) in the patient with pulmonary fibrosis.

The slope of the pressure-volume curve between two

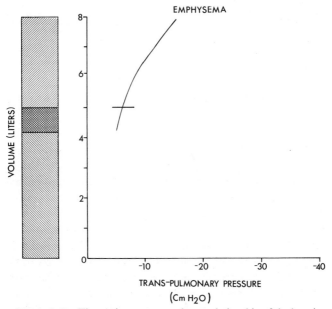

Figure 2–7. The static pressure–volume relationship of the lung in a patient with emphysema is graphed. Note that the functional residual capacity and total lung capacity are increased in comparison with the healthy individual shown in Figure 2–6, that the curve is shifted upward and to the left, and that the slope of the curve is greater, i.e., the compliance ($\Delta V / \Delta P$) is higher.

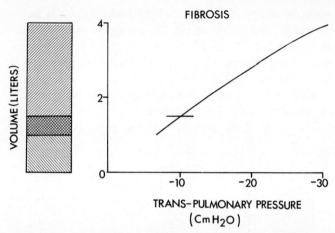

Figure 2–8. Depicted is the static pressure–volume relationship of the lung in a patient with pulmonary fibrosis. Note that the functional residual capacity and total lung capacity are reduced in comparison with the healthy individual in Figure 2–6, that the curve is shifted downward and to the right, and that the slope of the curve is less, i.e., the compliance ($\Delta V / \Delta P$) is lower.

particular volumes is the compliance of the lung over that volume. However, because the pressure-volume curve of the lung is not linear, it is clear that any single value of compliance is virtually meaningless, for the value depends on the lung volume at which it was determined. If a subject was breathing near TLC the lung appears to be stiffer (i.e., compliance is low) than that of another person breathing near his FRC, even though the intrinsic elastic properties of the lungs of both individuals may be identical. Thus it is important to evaluate the static pressure-volume relationships over the entire vital capacity and to know the lung volume at which the subject is breathing (i.e., functional residual capacity).

Dynamic Compliance

When the compliance of the lungs is determined during breathing (i.e., the volume change during a breath is divided by the change in trans-pulmonary pressure from end-expiration to end-inspiration) it is called dynamic compliance (C_{dyn}). As will be indicated later, this determination, of itself, may not be indicative of the elastic properties of the lung. In addition, it is apparent that the compliance value obtained will depend on the lung volume at which the subject was breathing.

FLOW RESISTANCE

In addition to the elastic recoil of the lungs and the chest wall, the respiratory muscles encounter flow-resistive properties of the lungs and chest wall during breathing. Unlike the elastic resistance, which is proportional to lung volume and is uninfluenced by the rate at which lung volume is changing, the flow resistance is proportional to the rapidity with which lung volume is changing. In addition, flow resistance is influenced by lung elastic recoil pressure and therefore secondarily by the lung volume.

The amount of force that must be applied during breathing depends upon the amount of resistance to airflow through the upper airways and the tracheo-bronchial tree, the frictional resistance of tissues sliding over one another in the lung parenchyma and the chest wall, and the elastic resistance. A third type of flow resistance, inertia, that must be overcome during acceleration and deceleration of the gas or tissues, is also present, but is generally considered negligible. During inspiration the force required to overcome flow resistance is nor-

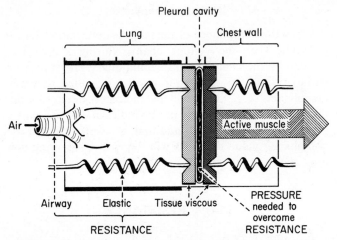

Figure 2–9. The resistances that must be overcome in order to move air into the lungs during breathing are illustrated. In addition to the elastic resistance offered by the two sets of springs, there is resistance to movement when the muscle contracts because of flow resistance in the airways and the sliding of tissues over one another. Thus the pressure in the pleural space that the muscles must develop is the sum of that required to overcome the elastic resistance of the lung to distention and the flow resistance.

mally provided by the respiratory muscles, while the elastic recoil of the lungs is sufficient to overcome gas and tissue flow resistance during expiration. During a forced and rapid expiration however, the elastic recoil of the lungs is insufficient to overcome the flow resistance and additional forces must be applied by contraction of the respiratory muscles.

In Figure 2–9 the mechanical analogue is again shown. In this case a nozzle (or airway) having a flow resistance as well as the frictional resistance developed by the plates sliding along the walls of the container has been depicted. Although the flow resistance is distributed in a much more complex fashion throughout the multibranched tracheobronchial tree and tissues, the model will allow us to demonstrate how it is possible to separate the flow-resistive and the elastic properties during breathing.

Figure 2–10 shows the excursions of "volume" and pressures during a "breath" produced in the model. As in the human, the pressure at the airway opening (mouth or nose) is atmospheric, whereas the pressure in the balloon (pleural space) varies. The upper curve illustrates the flow rate during breathing. By convention, inspiratory flow is plotted below and expiratory flow above the zero-flow line. The curve immediately below represents the change in volume, and the next curve down, the pressure in the balloon (the "intrapleural pressure"). The lowermost curve represents the pressure within the container (alveolar pressure). Since the frictional resistance is a small part of the flow resistance, this curve is a reflection of the resistance to airflow through the nozzle (airway resistance) and is depicted as the flow-resistive pressure.

From these traces of flow, volume, and pressure it is possible to separate the elastic resistance and the flow resistance of the lung at every instant during the "breath." The total pressure (P_t) applied is the sum of that required to overcome the elastic resistance (el) and the flow resistance (R).

$$P_t = P_{el} + P_R$$

Figure 2–10 indicates that at the extremes of the volume cycle (i.e., at the end of expiration and of inspiration)

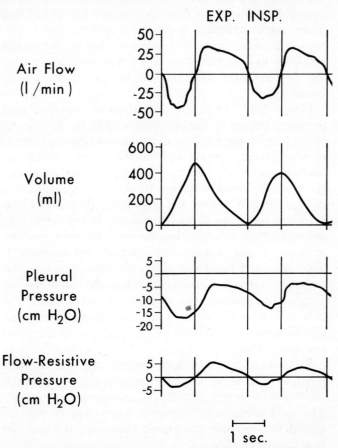

Figure 2–10. The relationship between pleural pressure, flow-resistive pressure, airflow, and volume is shown in the model. Note that the flow-resistive pressure is atmospheric at end expiration and end inspiration when there is no airflow. The compliance can be determined by dividing the volume change between these points by the change in pleural pressure.

there is no airflow, and the flow-resistive pressure passes through zero pressure at these points. In other words, at these instants all the pressure between the airway opening and the balloon (pleural space) is being applied to the elastic resistance.

$$P_t = P_{el}$$

The dynamic compliance can be calculated by dividing the volume change between the two points of zero flow by the change in applied or pleural pressure between these instants:

$$\text{Compliance} = \frac{\Delta \text{Volume}}{\Delta \text{Pressure}}$$

The elastic component of the total pressure at any point between end-inspiration and end-expiration during the breath is interpolated by assuming that the compliance is constant over the range of movement during the tidal volume. (This is equivalent to saying that for every mm change in the length of the spring or each ml of volume change in the container or lung, there is a fixed increment in elastic pressure.) Then at any volume in the cycle:

$$\Delta P_{el} = \frac{\Delta \text{Volume}}{\text{Compliance}}$$

Since, at any instant in the respiratory cycle, $P_R = P_t - P_{el}$, it is therefore possible to calculate the pressure necessary to overcome the flow resistance at any moment during the respiratory cycle.

By measuring the rate of airflow at the same instant as

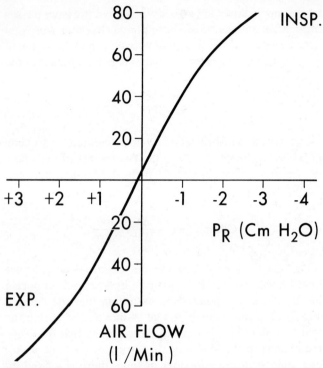

Figure 2–11. The relationship between flow-resistive pressure and airflow in a healthy individual is shown. The resistance to airflow, $(R) = P_R/Flow$, is about 1.5 cm H_2O/ℓ/sec at a flow rate of 1.0 ℓ/sec in healthy individuals.

that for which the flow-resistive pressure was calculated, a pressure-flow plot can be derived. This is illustrated in Figure 2–11 in which inspiration is shown in the upper right and expiration in the lower left quadrants. It will be noted that the pressure change is linearly related to the airflow up to a certain point, after which there is a dis-

proportionate increase in the pressure required to produce a further increase in airflow. The linear portion of
the curve is due to laminar resistance, and the deviation
from the straight line relationship is due to the development of turbulent resistance.

Flow resistance (R) is defined as the pressure required to produce a given rate of airflow and is expressed

$$R = \frac{P_R}{Flow}$$

in units of cm H_2O/ℓ/sec.

Although continuous measurement of alveolar pressure is not feasible in practice, it can be appreciated that
it is not really necessary because the pressure required
to overcome flow resistance can be determined from
simultaneous recordings of changes in lung volume,
airflow, and trans-pulmonary pressure during breathing,
all of which are obtainable in patients. In healthy individuals the flow resistance ranges between 1.0 and
3.0 cm H_2O/ℓ/sec of airflow, and only about one tenth
of the resistance at a flow rate of 1 ℓ/sec is due to tur-
bulence. In patients suffering from conditions such as
bronchitis, or during acute asthmatic attacks, the resistance to airflow may be 10 to 15 times that seen in
healthy individuals.

FLOW RESISTANCE AND LUNG VOLUME

The resistance to airflow varies with lung volume, and
is less at higher lung volumes (Fig. 2–12). This is because, as lung volume increases and pleural pressure becomes more subatmospheric, those parts of the tracheo-

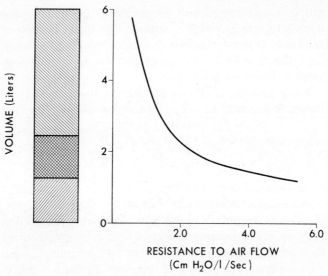

Figurr 2–12. The graph shows the relationship between resistance to airflow and lung volume in a normal individual. The airways are more distended at higher lung volumes because the transpulmonary pressure is more negative, so that the flow resistance is lower at high lung volumes.

bronchial tree that are exposed to the pleural pressure increase in size as a result of the increase in transbronchial pressure. Clearly then, determination of airflow resistance requires knowledge of the absolute lung volume at which measurements were made.

It is important to point out that measurements of airway resistance and indices of flow resistance derived from a forced vital capacity such as $FEV_{1.0}$ predominantly reflect resistance to airflow in airways that are greater than 2 mm in diameter. Although airways smaller than 2 mm in diameter are far more numerous and provide a total cross sectional area for airflow that is many times that of the central airways, the resistance in these small peripheral airways constitutes less than 20 per cent of the total airway resistance. The flow through the individual peripheral airways is small, and there is very little pressure drop across them. As a result, significant disease of the small peripheral airways may seriously impair ventilation of the air spaces distal to them, and yet total airway resistance may be little altered. Fortunately, there are now a number of determinations that are thought to reflect alterations in the peripheral airways. These are based on the interrelationships between lung elastic recoil and flow resistance in the peripheral airways.

UPSTREAM RESISTANCE

During a forced inspiration, the maximal airflow rate achieved at every lung volume is dependent to a major extent on the muscular effort developed. On the other hand, during a forced expiration, the maximal flow rate achieved at a particular lung volume is related to effort (pressure) only up to a certain point. Beyond this, increased effort does not lead to a higher flow rate, and may even be associated with a slight reduction in flow rate. This phenomenon can be observed by performing a series of active expirations of increasing force at a particular lung volume. If the airflow rates are plotted against the corresponding trans-pulmonary pressures, an **isovolume pressure-flow curve** is obtained. Figure 2–13 illustrates examples of such curves at three different lung volumes. At high lung volumes the airways are widely open so that very high flows can be achieved, just as in a forced inspiration the flow rate appears to be related to the amount of effort exerted. At lung volumes

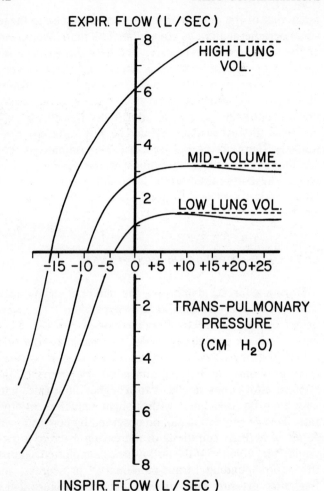

Figure 2–13. Isovolume pressure–flow curves obtained in a normal subject at three levels of lung inflation are illustrated. At high lung volume, maximum expiratory flow increases with increasing effort. At lower lung volumes increasing pressure raises the airflow rate up to a maximum, and further effort produces no further increase in flow, presumably because of airways compression (see Figure 2–14).

below 75 per cent of the vital capacity, on the other hand, highest flow rate ($\dot{V}_{max}$) is not achieved by the greatest trans-pulmonary pressure. The flow rate increases with effort only up to a certain point, beyond which further effort or greater driving pressure does not lead to a higher flow rate.

Since, as we have already seen, Flow Resistance (R) = Pressure/Flow, it is clear that after $\dot{V}_{max}$ has been achieved the resistance to airflow must rise in direct proportion to driving pressure. This rise in airflow resistance that occurs at each lung volume is due to dynamic compression of the airways.

This concept of dynamic compression of the airways is particularly important, and may be better understood with the aid of another model such as that shown in Figure 2–14. Here the pleural pressure (P_{pl}), which reflects the amount of effort exerted during the forced expiration, is 20 cm H_2O, and the recoil pressure of the lung (P_{el}) at this volume is assumed to be 10 cm H_2O. In this circumstance the pressure in the alveoli (P_{alv}), which is the sum of the elastic recoil pressure of the lung and the pleural pressure, is 30 cm H_2O.

It will be seen that the pressure in the airway diminishes from the alveolus (30 cm H_2O) to the airway opening (0 cm H_2O). Clearly then, there must be a point between the alveolus and the airway opening where the airway pressure is equal to the pleural pressure. This point in the airway has been called the **equal pressure point** (EPP). In the airways downstream from the EPP (i.e., between it and the mouth) the pressure is less than the pleural pressure, so these airways are subject to compression or closure during a forced expiration. The greater the amount of effort or driving pressure that is generated, the higher the pleural pressure and the more these downstream airways will be compressed. For air-

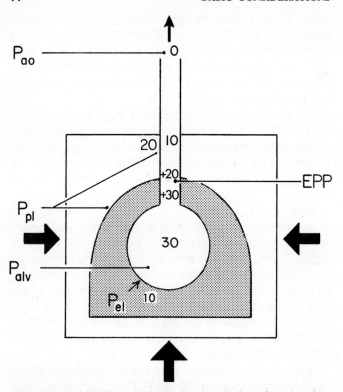

Figure 2–14. The forces acting in the chest during a forced expiratory effort are depicted. The heavy arrows indicate compression of the thorax by contraction of the expiratory muscles. P_{pl} equals the pleural pressure, in this case 20 cm H_2O. P_{el} equals elastic recoil pressure of the lung, in this case 10 cm H_2O. P_{alv} equals pressure in the alveolus = P_{pl} (20) + P_{el} (10) = 30 cm H_2O. Note that the pressure in the airways drops from the alveolar pressure (30 cm H_2O) to the mouth or P_{ao} (or atmospheric pressure). EPP indicates the "equal pressure point," i.e., the point in the airway at which the intramural and extramural pressures are equal, in this case 20 cm H_2O. Farther downstream from the equal pressure point, toward the airway opening, there is a transmural pressure tending to narrow or close the airway.

ways upstream from the EPP (between it and the alveoli) the driving pressure is the difference between the pressure in the alveoli and the airway pressure at the EPP (i.e., $P_{alv} - P_{pl}$) or, in other words, the elastic recoil pressure of the lungs (P_{el}). Since, as we have seen, it is possible to determine the relationship between the lung elastic recoil pressure and lung volume, a plot of the relationship between the pressures and maximum expiratory flow rates ($\dot{V}_{max}$) at equivalent volumes provides us with the pressure-flow relationships of the upstream segment of the airways and, in addition, the upstream resistance (R_{us}) can be calculated (Fig. 2–15).

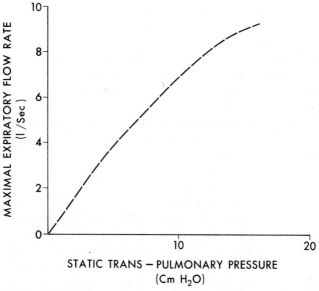

Figure 2–15. The graph shows the relationship between the transpulmonary pressure (lung elastic recoil) and the maximal expiratory flow rate ($\dot{V}_{max}$), i.e., the resistance to airflow in the upstream segment of the airways.

$$R_{us} = \frac{P_{el}}{\dot{V}_{max}}$$

MAXIMUM EXPIRATORY FLOW RATE

This formula indicates that the $\dot{V}_{max}$ at any lung volume is dependent on the relationship between the lung elastic recoil and the resistance to airflow in the airways upstream from the EPP.

$$\dot{V}_{max} = \frac{P_{el}}{R_{us}}$$

It is generally considered that the $\dot{V}_{max}$, at least at lung volumes below 60 per cent of the vital capacity, may be a sensitive indicator of changes in elastic recoil pressure or of the resistance of small airways. Clearly $\dot{V}_{max}$ could be lower than expected when the upstream resistance is increased (i.e.. airway narrowing), the driving pressure is reduced (i.e., loss of elastic recoil), or when both disturbances are present. As a corollary to this, it should be clear that if the driving pressure at a particular lung volume were greater than expected (for instance in pulmonary fibrosis), the $\dot{V}_{max}$ might be greater than expected if there has not been a proportionate increase in the upstream resistance.

Thus disease of the more peripheral units may be recognized by an increase in upstream resistance. On the other hand, disease of the peripheral units may not be sufficient to elevate the upstream resistance significantly and yet may alter the distribution of gas, particularly when the respiratory rate is rapid. This may be recognized by determination of the dynamic compliance of the lung at varying respiratory rates.

FREQUENCY DEPENDENCE OF COMPLIANCE

The distribution of gas to individual peripheral lung units is dependent on the impedance to inflation of each unit, and is affected by the product of the compliance of the unit and the flow resistance of the airway leading to it. This is analogous to the product of the resistance and capacitance of an electrical circuit, and is called its **time constant** (RC). Non-uniformly distributed alterations of the elastic or flow-resistive properties of the peripheral lung units, i.e., inequality of time constants in the lung, influence the distribution of gas in the lungs and affect the measurement of compliance during breathing (i.e., dynamic compliance).

An example of this phenomenon is shown in Figure 2–16, in which two lungs are depicted for simplicity. In the normal situation the compliance and flow resistance are the same in both units (Fig. 2–16A); here a change in pleural pressure of 5 cm H_2O is associated with an inspiration of 500 ml into each lung, so that the compliance is 1.0/5 or .200 ℓ/cm H_2O. In Figure 2–16B the elastic recoil of the two lungs is similar, but flow resistance is increased in one of the airways. In this circumstance, the measured compliance would probably not be different if the tidal volume were inhaled exceedingly slowly because flow resistance would be minimal, and the major impedance to changes in volume in the two lungs will be the elastic recoil. On the other hand, if the same tidal volume change were produced very rapidly, the rate of airflow would be high in the airways and the principal impedance to volume change would be flow-resistive.

Since the flow-resistances of the two lungs are markedly dissimilar, the lungs will not share equally in the total volume change, and the majority of the change will take

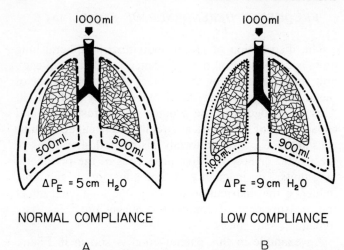

Figure 2–16. Represented is the effect of a local airway obstruction on the pressure–volume relationship of two lungs that have the same elastic properties when 1000 ml of air is inhaled during breathing. When there is no difference in flow resistance, the major impedance to lung distention is the elastic resistance, and both lungs share the inspired volume equally. When there is local obstruction, particularly at rapid respiratory rates (high flow rates), the major impedance will be flow-resistive, the inspired volume will be distributed unequally, and the calculated compliance of the lungs will be lower.

place through the airway with the lower resistance. Thus a greater pressure will have to be exerted in order to bring in the same tidal volume. A similar finding would occur if the resistance to air flow was similar in both units, but the compliance were dissimilar. The faster the breathing rate, the lower will be the measured compliance. In the example shown, virtually all of the volume change at extremely high frequencies could take place in and out of one unit, and if this were to occur, the calculated compliance would be approximately one half that obtained during exceedingly slow breathing.

In healthy lungs the measured compliance does not change even though the respiratory rate is increased to about 60/min (Fig. 2–17). This is remarkable, since that means that the distribution of elastic and flow-resistive properties of the lung units is such that the time constants, and therefore the distribution of inspired gas, is the same over this range of respiratory rate. A fall in lung compliance with increasing respiratory rate, as is

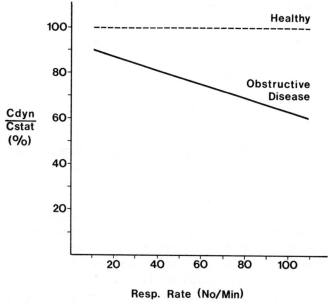

Figure 2–17. The effect of increased respiratory frequency on the calculated lung compliance in a healthy subject and in a patient with obstruction to airflow is shown. The patient with airflow obstruction demonstrates frequency-dependence of compliance.

also shown in Figure 2–17, is called **frequency-dependence** of compliance. The finding of a frequency dependence of compliance indicates an abnormal distribution of ventilation in the lungs. When this is found in a patient in whom lung compliance and airway resistance appear normal, it is thought to reflect alterations in the peripheral lung units.

WORK OF BREATHING

Till now we have talked about the various resistances offered by the respiratory apparatus. This subject is important clinically because the respiratory muscles must perform work in order to overcome the mechanical impedances to respiration offered by the lung and the chest wall during breathing.

MECHANICAL WORK

Work is usually defined as force acting through a distance and is expressed as dynes/cm. In the respiratory system it is convenient to consider the product of pressure and volume, which also has the units of work dynes/cm^2 × cm^3. The work performed to overcome elastic resistance during a breath can be determined by plotting the relationship between the volume and the elastic component of the trans-pulmonary pressure during a single inspiration. This is shown in Figure 2–18A, in which the shaded area represents the work performed against elastic forces. In Figure 2–18B, the work required to overcome the resistance to airflow during that breath has been added. It can be seen that

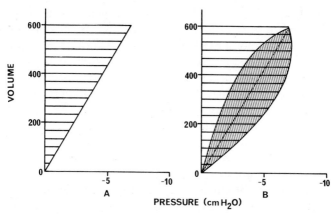

Figure 2–18. The mechanical work of breathing necessary to over-come elastic resistance is shown in A. In B the work required to over-come flow resistance is added. The expiratory portion of the flow resistance work loop falls within the triangle that represents elastic work, indicating that expiration is passive and brought about by the elastic force of the lung, which was built up during inspiration. Thus the total work performed during inspiration is the sum of the elastic work and that required to overcome inspiratory flow resistance.

this is represented by the area between the line indicative of the total pressure and that required to overcome the elastic properties. During a quiet expiration, the potential energy stored in the elastic structures during inspiration is normally sufficient to accomplish the work necessary to overcome flow resistance during expiration. When the mechanical properties of the respiratory apparatus are altered by disease, or during a forceful expiration, additional expiratory mechanical work is necessary. In healthy individuals, therefore, during quiet breathing, the total mechanical work per breath is equal to the sum of work performed to overcome the elastic properties and the flow resistance, and the work per minute is the work per breath times the respiratory rate. In healthy individuals the total mechanical work performed has been estimated to be approximately 0.3 to 0.7 kg-m/min, with about two thirds of this being done against elastic forces.

Figure 2–19 illustrates the effect of alterations of the mechanical properties of the lung on the mechanical work of breathing. The pressure-volume plot seen when the flow-resistive work increases (as in bronchial asthma) is illustrated in Figure 2–19A. Under these circumstances, the elastic energy stored during inspiration is insufficient to produce airflow during expiration, and the expiratory muscles must perform additional work. The effect of an increase in elastic resistance of the lungs

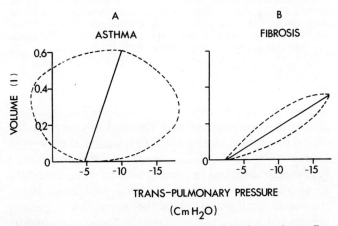

Figure 2–19.   The mechanical work of breathing in a patient suffering from bronchial asthma is shown in A, and that in a patient suffering from pulmonary fibrosis is shown in B. Note that the flow resistance loop falls outside of the elastic work area in the patient with asthma. Thus additional work was necessary to overcome flow resistance during expiration in this patient.

(as in pulmonary fibrosis) on mechanical work is shown in Figure 2–19*B*. The work required to overcome flow resistance is only slightly altered, but much more work must be performed in order to overcome the high elastic resistance of the "stiff lungs."

Mechanical Work and Alveolar Ventilation

The work of breathing can influence the pattern of breathing, and thereby the amount of ventilation actually taking part in gas exchange. Figure 2–20*A* illustrates that, for any given alveolar ventilation, there is an optimum respiratory rate and tidal volume at which the total mechanical work of breathing is minimal. When the respiratory rate is less than the optimum, the flow-resistive work is less but larger tidal volumes are necessary to achieve a given alveolar ventilation, and the amount of work required to overcome the elastic resistance increases considerably. When the respiratory rate is greater than the optimum, the total ventilation must increase if the same alveolar ventilation is to be maintained because more ventilation is wasted per minute when the tidal volume is smaller. Although the amount of work required to overcome elastic resistance is less, the flow-resistive work will increase, roughly in proportion to the increase in respiratory rate.

When the mechanical properties of the respiratory apparatus are altered by disease, the respiratory pattern is frequently altered accordingly. If the elastic resistance increases, as in pulmonary fibrosis or kyphoscoliosis, the curve representing the relationship between respiratory rate and mechanical work required to overcome elastic resistance is shifted upward and the work is minimal at an increased frequency. In these patients,

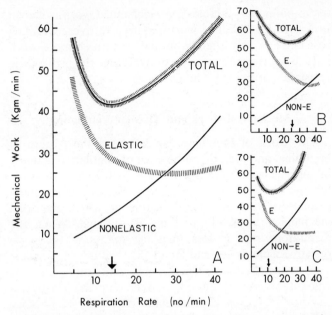

Figure 2–20. Depicted is the effect of respiratory rate on the mechanical work of breathing for a particular alveolar ventilation: normally (A), when the elastic work is increased (B), and when the non-elastic work is increased (C). The arrows indicate the respiratory rate at which total work is minimal.

then, the respirations tend to become rapid and shallow (Fig. 2–20B). Conversely, when the flow resistance increases, as in bronchial obstruction, the curve representing the relationship between respiratory rate and flow-resistive work is shifted upward and the work is minimal at a lower frequency. In these patients the respirations tend to become slower and deeper (Fig. 2–20C).

Mechanical Work and Oxygen Cost

In order to perform the work necessary to overcome the mechanical resistances encountered during breathing, the respiratory muscles require oxygen. Figure 2–21 illustrates that the oxygen consumption increases about 1 ml/ℓ of ventilation (range is 0.3 to 1.8 ml) when ventilation is increased up to about 60 ℓ/min in healthy individuals. At very high ventilations, the oxygen consumption increases considerably and may become a significant proportion of the total body oxygen consumption.

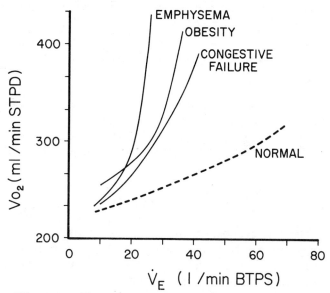

Figure 2–21. The change in oxygen consumption associated with increases in ventilation in a normal subject and patients with respiratory insufficiency is shown. In the patients, small increases in ventilation are associated with marked increases in oxygen consumption, i.e., the oxygen cost of breathing is higher.

Figure 2–21 also shows that the oxygen cost of breathing is increased in many respiratory disorders. In the patient suffering from emphysema, the oxygen cost, even at low ventilations, may be 4 to 10 times that of the healthy individual. In addition it should be noted that the oxygen consumption increases disproportionately at very low ventilations in patients with respiratory insufficiency. In such patients, then, any activity that necessitates an increase in ventilation will be associated with increased oxygen requirements of the respiratory apparatus, which may play an important role in limiting exercise tolerance. In fact, it has been suggested that exercise tolerance may depend on the relationship between the total body oxygen uptake and the oxygen requirements of the respiratory apparatus. According to this hypothesis the oxygen uptake during exercise may be inadequate to meet the needs of both the respiratory muscles and exercising non-respiratory muscles. As a result, one or the other group of muscles (or both) must go into oxygen debt so that exercise is limited.

The relationship between mechanical work and energy consumption represents the efficiency of a system:

$$\text{Efficiency } (\%) = \frac{\text{mechanical work}}{\text{energy cost}}$$

The energy cost of the respiratory muscles during breathing has been esimated to be between 6 and 24 kg m/min. Thus the efficiency of the respiratory apparatus in healthy individuals would appear to be low (between 2 and 10 per cent) when compared with that of other muscles. Although the exact mechanism has not been elucidated, it would appear that the efficiency of the respiratory apparatus is even lower in patients with cardiorespiratory disease.

SELF-ASSESSMENT

1. In 3 patients the following measurements were made

Measurement	Patient A	Patient B	Patient C
Pleural pressure at end-expiration	-2 cm H_2O	-3 cm H_2O	-4 cm H_2O
Pleural pressure at end-inspiration (inspired volume 800 ml)	-4 cm H_2O	-7 cm H_2O	-14 cm H_2O
Pleural pressure during mid-inspiration (inspired volume 400 ml)	-7 cm H_2O	-10 cm H_2O	-10 cm H_2O
Airflow rate at mid-inspiration	1.0 ℓ/sec	0.5 ℓ/sec	2.0 ℓ/sec

a. For each patient give
   (1) Lung compliance A _____
                        B _____
                        C _____
   (2) Flow resistance A _____
                        B _____
                        C _____
   (3) Likely diagnosis A _____
                        B _____
                        B _____

b. For each of the following parameters, indicate in each patient whether they would be anticipated to be _____
   (1) high.   (2) low.   (3) normal.

	A	B	C
FEV$_{1.0}$/FVC ratio			
Residual volume			
Functional residual capacity			
Total lung capacity			

2. When the lungs become fibrosed

  a. The force necessary to overcome elastic resistance is ___
     (1) high.   (2) low.   (3) unchanged.

  b. The force necessary to overcome non-elastic resistance
     is _____
     (1) high.   (2) low.   (3) unchanged.

  c. The respiratory rate is _____
     (1) slow.   (2) fast.   (3) unchanged.

  d. The tidal volume is _____
     (1) low.   (2) high.   (3) unchanged.

  e. Vital capacity is _____
     (1) normal.   (2) low.   (3) greater than normal.

  f. $\dot{V}_{max}$ 50 is _____ expected.
     (1) lower than   (2) higher than   (3) unchanged from

  g. Total lung capacity is _____
     (1) reduced.   (2) increased.   (3) unchanged.

3. With assumption of the supine position

  a. The resting level moves to _____
     (1) a more inspiratory position.
     (2) a more expiratory position.
     (3) is unchanged.

  b. The expiratory reserve volume _____
     (1) increases.   (2) decreases.   (3) is unchanged.

  c. The inspiratory capacity _____
     (1) increases.   (2) decreases.   (3) is unchanged.

    d. The end-expiratory intrapleural pressure is _____
       (1) more negative. (2) less negative. (3) unchanged.

4. At normal end-inspiration

    a. Intrapleural pressure is _____ atmospheric pressure.
       (1) less than   (2) more than   (3) equal to

    b. Intra-alveolar pressure is _____ atmospheric pressure.
       (1) less than   (2) more than   (3) equal to

    c. Intrapleural pressure is _____ intra-alveolar pressure.
       (1) less than   (2) more than   (3) equal to

    d. Intra-alveolar pressure is _____ that at the end of
       expiration.
       (1) higher than   (2) lower than   (3) equal to

5. During a forced expiratory effort intra-alveolar pressure
   is _____ intrapleural pressure.
       (1) less than   (2) more than   (3) equal to

6. With a constant minute ventilation, if an increase in frequency occurs

    a. dead space ventilation is _____
       (1) increased.   (2) decreased.   (3) unchanged.

    b. elastic work/breath is _____
       (1) increased.   (2) decreased.   (3) unchanged.

    c. flow resistance is _____
       (1) increased.   (2) decreased.   (3) unchanged.

7. In a normal subject, change in volume of the lung (ΔV) is
   plotted against a corresponding change in trans-pulmonary
   pressure (ΔTPP). Measurement is by means of an intra-
   esophageal balloon during a single quiet breath at rest.
   Results are shown in Figure 2–22.

    a. The compliance of the lung is represented on the dia-
       gram by _____

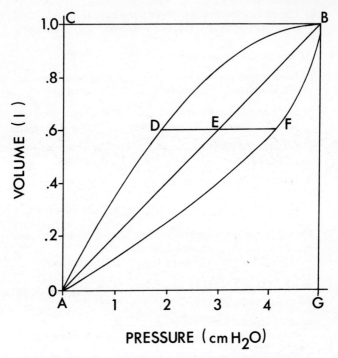

Figure 2–22. The graph illustrates the relationship between change in trans-pulmonary pressure and volume during a single breath.

  (1) $\Delta V \times \Delta TPP$.   (2) $\Delta V/\Delta TPP$.   (3) $\Delta TPP/\Delta V$.
  (4) Δ Flow$/\Delta TPP$.   (5) $\Delta TPP/\Delta$ Flow.
  (6) none of these.

b. The airway plus tissue resistance of the lung is represented by _____
  (1) $\Delta V \times \Delta TPP$.   (2) $\Delta V/\Delta TPP$.   (3) $\Delta TPP/\Delta V$.
  (4) Δ Flow$/\Delta TPP$.   (5) $\Delta TPP/\Delta$ Flow.
  (6) none of these.

c. The total work done on the lung during a breath is equal
   to the area of _____
   (1) Figure ABCA.   (2) Figure AGBCA.
   (3) Loop AFBDA.   (4) Figure AFBCA.
   (5) Figure ADBCA.   (6) Figure AEBFA.

d. Increasing the frequency of breathing and maintaining
   the size of the breath will cause the area enclosed by the
   pressure-volume loop AFBDA to be _____
   (1) increased.   (2) decreased.   (3) unchanged.

e. Under these circumstances, the mechanical work per
   breath done on the lungs will be _____
   (1) increased.   (2) decreased.   (3) unchanged.

f. The mechanical work per minute will be _____
   (1) increased.   (2) decreased.   (3) unchanged.

Chapter 3

PULMONARY VENTILATION, BLOOD FLOW, AND GAS EXCHANGE

As we have learned, gas is exchanged between the alveolar air and the pulmonary capillary blood. Oxygen moves from the alveolus into the pulmonary capillary blood, and carbon dioxide enters the alveoli from the blood. Under normal circumstances the gas tensions of the blood that leaves the pulmonary capillaries are virtually in equilibrium with the gas tensions of the alveolar air; the P_{O_2} is about 100 torr and the P_{CO_2} about 40 torr (Fig. 3–1). However, even in young healthy individuals

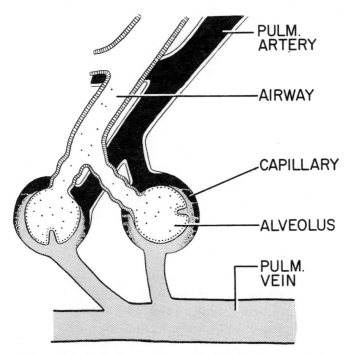

PULM. ARTERY

AIRWAY

CAPILLARY

ALVEOLUS

PULM. VEIN

Figure 3–1. "Ideal" gas exchange. In this situation not only has blood traversing the two lung units come into complete diffusion equilibrium with the alveolar gas, but each unit contributes to the mixed alveolar gas the same proportion of gas that it contributes to the mixed arterial blood.

the arterial P_{O_2} is about 10 torr less than the mixed alveolar (or end-capillary) P_{O_2} because the distribution of ventilation and perfusion throughout the lung are not perfectly matched. Some of the blood perfuses poorly ventilated areas of lung and is poorly oxygenated so that it acts as though it has bypassed alveoli. When this blood is added to the blood that has left well ventilated alveoli it causes a fall in the oxygen tension. On the other hand, the admixture of blood from poorly ventilated alveoli has much less impact on the P_{CO_2} than it does on the P_{O_2}, and the arterial P_{CO_2} is about 40 torr.

When the difference between the P_{O_2} in the alveoli and the arterial blood increases, or the arterial P_{O_2} is lower than normal (with or without an abnormal P_{CO_2}) gas exchange is abnormal. Although an abnormality of gas exchange can be the result of several disturbances, mismatching between ventilation and blood flow in the lungs accounts for the majority of the abnormalities of gas exchange; and alveolar hypoventilation, right to left shunts, or diffusion defects are encountered to a much lesser extent.

VENTILATION

The absolute quantity of air breathed normally is about 6 or 7 liters per minute. Practically speaking, however, it is the portion of the air we breathe that takes part in the exchange of gases between the blood and the alveoli that is important. Some of the air that fills the parts of the respiratory system that serve as a conducting airway (i.e., the dead space) is wasted, and does not take part in gas exchange (physiologic dead space).

DEAD SPACE

The mouth, nose, pharynx, larynx, trachea, bronchi, and the bronchioles are collectively called the anatomic dead space. However, as pointed out earlier the dead space is really a physiologic concept, and can be considered the volume of the inspired gas that does not take part in gas exchange. Actually, the ventilation of the dead space is really not that sharply divided from ventilation of the alveoli because over-ventilation of areas of lung, even though they are normally perfused, will contribute to the physiologic dead space.

In healthy young persons the physiologic dead space is approximately 150 ml at rest (i.e., about 20 to 30 per cent of each tidal volume). This is essentially wasted, so that only 70 to 80 per cent of each breath actually takes part in gas exchange. In patients suffering from pulmonary disease, the physiologic dead space is increased because of continued ventilation of alveoli whose perfusion is inadequate or even absent, or over-ventilation of other alveoli that are normally perfused. In these patients, therefore, a considerably greater proportion of each breath is wasted, and the amount taking part in gas exchange between the alveolar air and the pulmonary capillary blood is reduced.

ALVEOLAR VENTILATION

The air that takes part in gas exchange is called the alveolar ventilation. This all-important component of the air that is inhaled into the lungs can be influenced by several factors. Clearly a reduction or an increase in minute ventilation will decrease or increase the alveolar ventilation. However, even if the minute ventilation remains unchanged, the level of alveolar ventilation will be altered if there is a change in respiratory frequency (Table 3-1). Thus, with no change in minute ventilation, an increase in respiratory rate (which means that the tidal volume falls) will result in a fall in alveolar ventilation. A fall in alveolar ventilation as a result of rapid shallow respirations is frequently found in patients who are suffering from kyphoscoliosis or extreme obesity.

Table 3-2 demonstrates that if the physiologic dead space increases, the alveolar ventilation will also be reduced. In patients with emphysema, in which there is an increase in the number of alveoli that are ventilated but poorly perfused, the physiologic dead space is increased. The alveolar ventilation may not be reduced in these patients, however, because the tidal volume also increases. In fact, the increase in ventilation may even result in a rise in alveolar ventilation. However, because of the marked increase in work of breathing that the increased ventilation entails, many patients with chronic respiratory disease are unable to maintain their alveolar ventilation, and this has a deleterious effect on gas exchange.

Table 3-1 EFFECT OF RESPIRATORY RATE AND TIDAL VOLUME ON ALVEOLAR VENTILATION WHEN MINUTE VENTILATION AND DEAD SPACE ARE CONSTANT

$\dot{V}_E$ (ℓ/min)	V_D (ml)	V_T (ml)	f	$\dot{V}_A$ (ℓ/min)
8.0	150	1000	8	6.8
8.0	150	500	16	5.6
8.0	150	250	32	3.2

Table 3–2 EFFECT OF INCREASE IN DEAD SPACE ON ALVEOLAR VENTILATION WHEN MINUTE VENTILATION AND RESPIRATORY RATE ARE CONSTANT

$\dot{V}_E$ (ℓ/min)	V_D (ml)	V_T (ml)	f	$\dot{V}_A$ (ℓ/min)
8.0	150	500	16	5.6
8.0	200	500	16	4.8
8.0	250	500	16	4.0

The absolute level of the alveolar ventilation is not the major factor that determines whether or not it is adequate for gas exchange. Since the exchange of oxygen and carbon dioxide between the body and the environment is carried out by the alveolar ventilation, its adequacy must be judged in relation to the body's oxygen consumption and carbon dioxide production. In practice it is convenient to consider the adequacy of the alveolar ventilation in terms of its relationship to the metabolic carbon dioxide production. As we shall see, this relationship determines the alveolar and arterial P_{CO_2}. An analogous relationship can be derived between alveolar ventilation and the alveolar P_{O_2}.

In the steady state, the metabolic production of carbon dioxide by the body ($\dot{V}_{CO_2}$) is equal to the amount of carbon dioxide being eliminated by the alveoli, which in turn is simply the difference between the volumes of carbon dioxide entering and leaving the alveoli per unit time. Since only negligible amounts of CO_2 enter the alveoli in the inspired air, then

$$\dot{V}_{CO_2} = \dot{V}_A \times F_{A_{CO_2}}$$

where $\dot{V}_{CO_2}$ is the CO_2 production, $\dot{V}_A$ is the alveolar ventilation, and $F_{A_{CO_2}}$ is the concentration of CO_2 in the alveoli

and
$$F_{A_{CO_2}} = \frac{\dot{V}_{CO_2}}{\dot{V}_A}$$

This equation can be expressed in terms of P_{CO_2} rather than $F_{A_{CO_2}}$ as follows

$$P_{A_{CO_2}}(torr) = \frac{\dot{V}_{CO_2}(ml/min)}{\dot{V}_A (\ell/min)} \times 0.863$$

The factor 0.863 converts gas concentration to partial pressure or torr and also corrects for the CO_2 production being expressed as a dry gas volume at STPD, while the alveolar ventilation is expressed as a wet gas volume at BTPS.

Because the difference between the arterial P_{CO_2} and that of the mixed alveolar gas is usually very small, the arterial P_{CO_2} is utilized as a measure of the "effective" alveolar P_{CO_2} and the adequacy of the alveolar ventilation to cope with the metabolic production of carbon dioxide. This is not true of the arterial P_{O_2} and it is not a reliable measure of the alveolar P_{O_2} because it is influenced considerably by many other factors besides the alveolar ventilation. When the alveolar ventilation is insufficient to cope with a given CO_2 production, the alveolar (and arterial) P_{CO_2} will be higher than normal (i.e., >45 torr) and **alveolar hypoventilation** is present. Conversely, when the alveolar ventilation is greater than is necessary to cope with the CO_2 production, the alveolar (and arterial) P_{CO_2} will be lower than normal (i.e., <35 torr) and **alveolar hyperventilation** is present.

DISTRIBUTION OF VENTILATION

Radioactive techniques have demonstrated that, even in healthy individuals, more of the inspired air is distributed to the bottom of the lung than to the top of the lung when the subject is breathing normally (Fig. 3–2). This is because although the pleural pressure was discussed earlier as though it were the same everywhere in

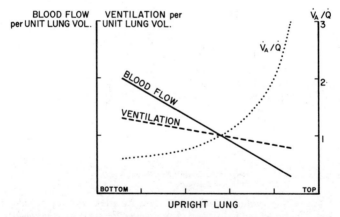

Figure 3–2. The graph shows the distribution of ventilation and blood flow in the upright lung. Both ventilation and blood flow are less at the top of the lung than at the bottom. The ventilation/perfusion ratios ($\dot{V}_A/\dot{Q}$) are very different at the top and bottom, the upper zones being overventilated in relation to their perfusion (high $\dot{V}_A/\dot{Q}$ ratio), whereas the lower regions are underventilated in relation to their perfusion (low $\dot{V}_A/\dot{Q}$ ratio).

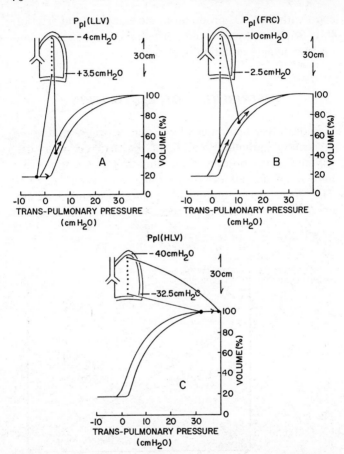

Figure 3–3. Graphs A through C show the effect of a pleural pressure gradient on the distribution of ventilation (the pressure is assumed to fall at a rate of 0.25 cm of water per cm of vertical distance). At low lung volumes (A) the pleural pressure at the base may exceed airway pressure so that this region is not ventilated and the initial part of inspiration is delivered to the apex of the lung. During an inspiration from FRC (B) air is distributed to the upper and lower parts of the lung. Because the pressures at the apex and base are taken to be −10 and

Legend continued on the opposite page

the chest, it isn't. At the top of the lung the force of gravity (weight of the lung) and the retractive force of the lung act in the same direction so that the pleural pressure is more negative than it is at the bottom of the lung, where the force of gravity and the retractive force of the lung act in opposite directions. It is generally considered that the pleural pressure increases by about 0.25 cm H_2O/cm of distance from the top to the bottom of the lungs. As a result of these differences in pleural pressure, areas near the top of the lung are more distended at FRC than others near the bottom of the lung. The difference between regions varies depending upon the lung volume, and, as is shown in Figure 3–3, because they are at different portions of their pressure-volume curves, the distribution of the inspired air to these regions will depend upon the lung volume at which one is breathing. If one were breathing at a low lung volume, the upper part of the lung would be ventilated more than the lower part (Fig. 3–3A). If breathing were to occur at near residual volume, the lower part of the lung would receive almost no ventilation at all because the airways in the dependent portions tend to close as a result of the higher pleural pressure. As indicated earlier, during ordinary breathing at FRC, the air spaces at the top of the lung

---

Figure 3–3. *Legend continued.* '2.5 cm of H_2O respectively, the two regions are on different parts of the pressure-volume curve, and the lung units at the base are smaller than those at the apex. On inspiration the lung units at the base have a greater change in volume than do those at the apex. At FRC, therefore, ventilation decreases with vertical distance up the lung. At high lung volumes (C) both upper and lower lung regions are on the flat part of the pressure–volume curve and exhibit changes in volume that correspond to changes in transpulmonary pressure.

tend to fill somewhat less on inspiration than those at the base (Fig. 3–3 *B*). On the other hand, at lung volumes close to TLC, both the upper and lower regions of the lung are on the flat part of the pressure-volume curve and the changes in volume, though minimal, tend to be similar (Fig. 3–3 *C*).

As we have seen in Chapter 2, the distribution of gas will be further altered if there are regional alterations of the mechanical resistances offered by the lung, the airways, or the extrapulmonary structures. This is demonstrated in Figure 3–4, which illustrates the effect of a local airway resistance on the distribution of inspired gas, as reflected by changes in the nitrogen concentration of the expired air following an inspiration of pure oxygen. Regional alterations of the elastic or tissue viscous resistance will alter the distribution of gas in a similar manner.

When there is no obstruction the inspired oxygen enters both lungs almost synchronously and equally, and expiration takes place in the same fashion (Fig. 3–4 *A*). The expired N_2 concentration curve illustrates what takes place during expiration. Initially there is no nitrogen in the expired air because only pure oxygen is exhaled from the dead space. The nitrogen concentration then rises in a curvilinear fashion as gas from the alveoli containing nitrogen is mixed with the oxygen from the dead space. The nitrogen concentration then virtually reaches a plateau as an equal amount of nitrogen is expired from each lung, the very slight rise in the plateau probably being due to sequential emptying of different areas of the lungs. The reader may recognize this as the plateau or Phase III of the single breath nitrogen washout curve from which closing volume is determined.

When the time constants of the various regions of the

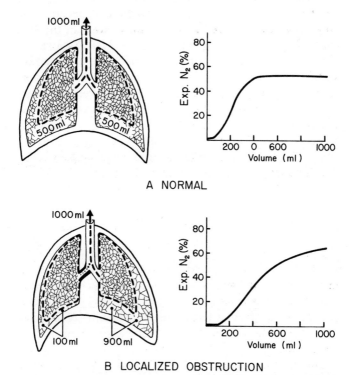

Figure 3–4. The effect of a localized airway obstruction on the distribution of air is depicted. Normally (A) air is distributed synchronously and equally, and expiration takes place in the same manner. As a result the nitrogen concentration reaches a virtual plateau. With localized airway obstruction (B), inspired oxygen predominantly moves into areas of lung which offer least resistance. During expiration air moves out of the unobstructed lung first and the asynchronous delivery of air results in a rising nitrogen concentration curve.

lung are non-uniformly distributed, such as occurs with localized obstruction to airflow, the inspired oxygen is asynchronously and unequally distributed because the oxygen moves preferentially into those areas of the lung that offer the least resistance (Fig. 3–4B). As a result, the nitrogen concentration in the unobstructed lung falls considerably because it is well diluted by the inhaled oxygen, while that in the obstructed lung remains high. During the ensuing expiration, gas moves out of the unobstructed lung first, and that from the obstructed lung is delayed. The asynchronous delivery of gas from the two lungs results in a rising nitrogen concentration curve (i.e., an increased slope of Phase III of the curve).

BLOOD FLOW

The main function of the pulmonary blood flow is to conduct mixed venous blood through the alveolar capillaries so that oxygen can be added and carbon dioxide removed. The absolute quantity of pulmonary blood flow is usually very similar to the absolute quantity of alveolar ventilation, the cardiac output being about 5 to 6 liters per minute.

The absolute amounts of ventilation and perfusion of the lungs in a period of time are important. To take it to an extreme, if ventilation were to stop altogether, the $P_{A_{O_2}}$ would fall and the $P_{A_{CO_2}}$ would rise sharply, and the blood leaving the lungs would continue to have a low oxygen tension and a high carbon dioxide tension. Similarly, if there were no blood flow, there would be no gas transfer and all the inspired gas would be wasted. However, even if the amount of alveolar ventilation and pulmonary blood flow were normal, hypoxemia might develop if the ratio of alveolar ventilation to perfusion were not uniform throughout the lungs.

We have seen that the distribution of ventilation in the lungs is not uniform even under normal circumstances. Let us now look at the distribution of the pulmonary blood flow, and how it matches up with the alveolar ventilation throughout the lung.

DISTRIBUTION OF BLOOD FLOW

As is shown in Figure 3–2, the blood flow is also less at the apex than at the base of the upright lung (subject sitting or standing). This is because the distribution of blood flow in the pulmonary vessels is profoundly influenced by the surrounding pressures. This effect is best demonstrated in a mechanical model in Figure 3–5. Here a collapsible tube representing a pulmonary capillary is surrounded by the alveolar pressure (P_{alv}). For flow to occur through the capillary, the perfusing pressure or pulmonary artery pressure must exceed all the pressures downstream, and there will be no flow if the capillary is closed off by a high alveolar pressure or elevated intraluminal pressure (P_c) resulting from an increased venous pressure (P_v). In other words, for a given pulmonary artery pressure the capillary will be narrowed, its resistance will increase, and flow will decrease if the alveolar pressure is elevated. The venous pressure will have no influence on flow as long as it is lower than the alveolar pressure. This arrangement has been likened to a waterfall in which the flow over the fall is independent of the height of the fall. However, if the venous pressure exceeds the alveolar pressure it will constitute an effective "back pressure" and interfere with blood flow.

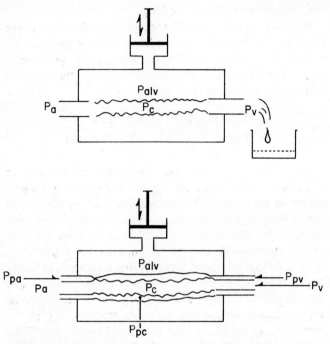

Figure 3–5. The upper model represents a small pulmonary vessel ("capillary") as a collapsible tube that is exposed to a variable extramural pressure analogous to alveolar pressure (P_{alv}). When the outflow pressure or "venous" pressure (P_v) is lower than P_{alv} it does not influence flow through the vessel. Flow will be determined by the dimension of the collapsible vessel and the inflow or "arterial" pressure (P_a). The dimension of the vessel is determined by its transmural pressure, i.e., the difference between its intraluminal and extraluminal pressures ($P_{alv} - P_c$). Only when P_v exceeds P_{alv} is it reflected "back," hence constituting an effective "back pressure" that influences flow.

The lower model has additional elements representing extramural forces acting on the "extra-alveolar" and "intra-alveolar" portions of the vessel. These include periarterial (P_{pa}) and perivenous (P_{pv}) forces such as interstitial pressure and smooth muscle tone. Pericapillary forces (P_{pc}) may include those related to the surface tension of the alveolar lining layer.

In Figure 3–6 the model has been expanded and the effect of gravity on the distribution of blood flow is depicted. Now the vascular bed of the lung is represented by a series of parallel vertical collapsible "capillaries" that are surrounded by the same alveolar pressure. The inflow and outflow channels are depicted as rigid tubes. The pulmonary artery pressure (P_{PA}) is represented by the inflow reservoir, which is kept filled to a height of

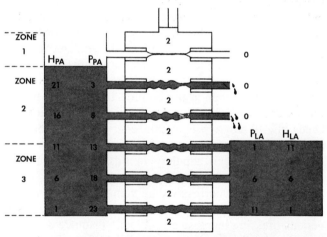

Figure 3–6. This model represents the pulmonary vascular bed. H_{PA} is height of inflow reservoir. P_{PA} represents pulmonary artery pressure. H_{LA} represents height of outflow reservoir. P_{LA} is left atrial pressure. Alveolar pressure (P_{alv}) equals 2 cm of water throughout the system. In zone 1, P_{alv} exceeds P_{PA} so there is no flow. In zone 2, P_{PA} exceeds P_{alv} so that flow varies with height, being greater near the bottom than at the top of the zone. In zone 3, P_{PA} exceeds P_{alv}, but P_{alv} is less than P_{LA}. Since P_{PA} and P_{LA} increase by equal amounts throughout this zone, flow through each channel in this zone is the same and does not vary with height.

23 cm H_2O above the "artery" at the lowest part of the lung. The height of the fluid in the outflow reservoir, which overflows when its fluid level is higher than 11 cm above the "vein" in the lowest part of the lung, is analogous to the left atrial pressure (P_{LA}).

An examination of this model indicates that the amount of blood flow depends on the height of the channel. In the upper part of the model (which in the lung has been called zone 1) the alveolar pressure of $+2$ cm H_2O exceeds the pulmonary artery pressure, which is 0, so that there is no blood flow. In the middle part (or zone 2) the pulmonary artery pressure exceeds the alveolar and left atrial pressures. In this zone, therefore, the amount of flow in each "capillary" depends on the gradient between the inflow pressure and the alveolar pressure ($P_{PA} - P_{alv}$), which in turn will vary with the height, being less at the top of the zone than at the bottom. In the lower part of the model (zone 3) the pulmonary artery pressure exceeds the alveolar pressure in every channel, but the alveolar pressure is less than the outflow pressure (P_{LA}). Flow through each capillary in this zone will be dependent on the difference between pulmonary artery pressure and the corresponding venous pressure ($P_{PA} - P_{LA}$). In this model, the pulmonary artery pressure and venous pressure increase equally with distance down the lung, so the driving pressure and therefore the flow in each channel is approximately the same, and does not vary with the height as it did in zone 2. In the lungs the same principles apply, but the inflow and outflow tubes are distensible rather than rigid, and they are affected by the transmural pressure acting on them. Unlike the model, the blood flow varies with height in zone 3 and is influenced by the resistance in the capillaries, which in turn is determined by their distensibility and the local transmural pressure.

From the model we can readily see that the distribution of blood flow will be altered when the pulmonary artery pressure and circulating blood volume are elevated (as might occur in heart failure) or when the pulmonary artery pressure and circulating blood volume are low (as occurs in severe hypotension and shock). Like the distribution of ventilation, the distribution of perfusion will be altered by changes in flow resistance and distensibility (compliance) of the pulmonary vessels in different regions in the lung, pulmonary vascular occlusion, embolization or thrombosis in pulmonary blood vessels, or obliteration of part of the pulmonary vasculature because of emphysema or fibrosis.

MATCHING OF VENTILATION AND BLOOD FLOW

As we have seen, even in a healthy person neither the distribution of the inspired gas nor the pulmonary blood flow are uniform throughout the lungs. From Figure 3–2 we can also see that the matching of blood and gas distribution ($\dot{V}_A/\dot{Q}$ ratios) is not uniform throughout the lung, even in healthy individuals, so that gas concentrations must differ from region to region. However, under normal circumstances this amount of mismatching is not sufficient to materially interfere with gas exchange, and the partial pressure of oxygen and carbon dioxide in the mixed arterial blood and the mixed alveolar gas are nearly the same.

VENOUS-ADMIXTURE-LIKE PERFUSION

When inadequately ventilated alveoli are well perfused as illustrated in Figure 3–7A or, in the extreme case, when alveoli receive no ventilation because they are full of exudate or the airway leading to them is blocked, but blood flow through their capillaries is excellent, then a low ventilation/perfusion ratio is present. Under such circumstances the blood flowing past the alveoli is only slightly aerated, if at all. This poorly aerated blood then mixes with fully "arterialized" blood coming from other pulmonary capillaries (**venous-admixture-like perfusion**), and, as a result, arterial hypoxemia and slight hypercapnia

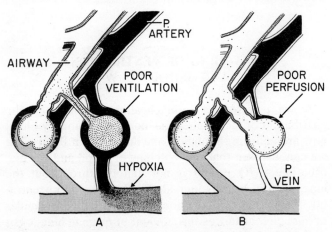

Figure 3–7. This figure shows the effect of alterations of ventilation/perfusion relationships on gas exchange. A, Low $\dot{V}_A/\dot{Q}$ areas contribute poorly oxygenated blood to the systemic circulation—an effect that is similar to that resulting from venous admixture (shunt). B, High $\dot{V}_A/\dot{Q}$ areas contribute gas to the mixed expired air, which is high in O_2 and low in CO_2 concentration—an effect similar to that resulting from an increase in dead space.

are present. Hypercapnia may not develop, however, if there is sufficient hyperventilation of the rest of the perfused alveoli. But hyperventilation of these alveoli adds only a limited amount of oxygen to the blood because of the shape of the oxyhemoglobin dissociation curve, so the arterial hypoxemia is not corrected to any significant degree.

DEAD-SPACE-LIKE VENTILATION

When the ventilation of alveoli is maintained but the blood perfusion is limited (Fig. 3–7B), or, in the extreme case, when there is no blood flow (as occurs when an embolus or thrombosis occludes a pulmonary artery), a high ventilation/perfusion ratio is present. This has been termed "alveolar dead space" or **dead-space-like ventilation** because the gas leaving such alveoli has taken little if any part in gas exchange, and its composition is much like the gas in the tracheobronchial tree. Adequate oxygenation and carbon dioxide elimination, as evidenced by the presence of normal arterial oxygen and carbon dioxide tensions, are frequent in the presence of excessive dead-space-like ventilation. However, the large amount of wasted ventilation means that the proportion of the ventilation that takes part in gas exchange, i.e., the alveolar ventilation, may be lower than required unless the total ventilation is increased. In the later stages of severe respiratory disease, the work of breathing may be so great (i.e., CO_2 production elevated) that a patient may be unable to increase his ventilation sufficiently to provide an adequate alveolar ventilation. Under these circumstances hypoxemia and hypercapnia will develop.

TRUE VENOUS ADMIXTURE OR SHUNT

The most gross example of mismatching that may be imagined is one in which some pulmonary capillary blood does not come into contact with any alveoli at all, so that mixed venous blood is added to arterialized blood (i.e., **true venous admixture** or a right-to-left shunt exists) (Fig. 3–8). Even in healthy persons approxi-

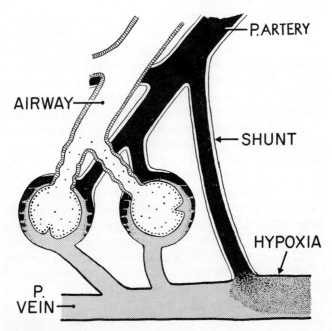

Figure 3–8. Poorly oxygenated blood, which does not come into contact with alveoli, is added to arterialized blood coming from ventilated alveoli. This is called true venous admixture or right-to-left shunt.

mately 2.5 per cent of the pulmonary blood flow enters the arterialized systemic circulation by means of the pulmonary veins and the thebesian and the bronchial veins, which empty into the left side of the heart. In some congenital heart lesions in which blood is shunted from the right to the left side, and in a pulmonary arteriovenous aneurysm in which blood is shunted from the pulmonary artery to the pulmonary veins, the amount of true venous admixture increases and considerable arterial hypoxemia may be present. In such conditions ventilation is generally increased as a result of the hypoxemic stimulus, and hypocapnia is common.

DIFFUSION OF GAS

The transfer of oxygen and carbon dioxide between the alveolar gas and the pulmonary capillary blood is entirely passive, and is brought about by diffusion. The rate of diffusion of a gas across the blood-gas barrier is dependent on its solubility in liquid, its density, the partial pressure difference between the alveolar air and the blood, and the surface area that is available for diffusion. Even though it is a larger molecule than oxygen, the solubility of carbon dioxide is almost 25 times as great, and it diffuses about 20 times more rapidly between air and blood than oxygen. For this reason the diffusion of carbon dioxide from the pulmonary capillaries to the alveoli is never a clinical problem.

A diffusion abnormality for oxygen is present if the capillary blood fails to achieve equilibrium with alveolar gas during its transit past the alveolus (Fig. 3–9). Contrary to earlier beliefs, an impaired diffusion of oxygen from the alveolar air to the pulmonary capillary blood is

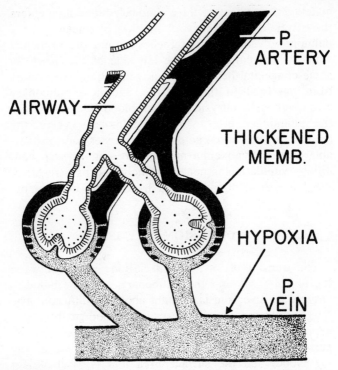

Figure 3–9. The effect of a diffusion abnormality for oxygen on gas exchange is shown. The end-capillary blood oxygen does not achieve equilibrium with alveolar gas.

seldom the primary cause of a low arterial oxygen tension. With the possible exception of a relatively rare group of patients who have a specific type of alveolar disorder, arterial hypoxemia in pulmonary disease, even when it is severe, is due to a mismatching of ventilation and perfusion in most situations.

SELF-ASSESSMENT

1. The lung of an upright subject is about 35 cm long from top to bottom, and the pulmonary artery pressure averages 12 cm H_2O.

   a. The intrapleural pressure near the top of the upright lung is _____ at the bottom.
   (1) greater than   (2) less than   (3) the same as

   b. At residual volume the alveolar dimensions at the bottom of the lung would consequently be ____ at the top.
   (1) greater than   (2) less than   (3) the same as

   c. The blood flow to the apex of the lung is _____ at the base.
   (1) greater than   (2) less than   (3) the same as

   d. The effect of increasing alveolar pressure by 5 mm Hg on the distribution of blood in the lung is to _____
   (1) increase the size of "zone 1."
   (2) cause complete cessation of blood flow through the entire lung.
   (3) increase the blood flow to the apical zone of the lung.
   (4) decrease the blood flow to the basal zone of the lung.

2. A high ventilation/perfusion ratio in a group of alveoli implies

   a. perfusion of poorly ventilated areas.
   b. ventilation of poorly perfused areas.
   c. venous-admixture-like perfusion.
   d. dead-space-like ventilation.

3. In a subject breathing room air (B.P. = 747 torr), P_{aO_2} was 70 torr. When the $P_{A_{O_2}}$ was 100 torr and $P_{C_{O_2}}$ was 99 torr, these findings indicate that the gas exchange defect is due to _____

   a. hypoventilation.
   b. anemic hypoxia.

c. venous admixture.
d. none of the above.

4. If the two lungs of an individual share the tidal volume equally after the artery to one lung is ligated

    a. The physiologic dead space would be ＿＿＿＿＿ that measured at the same tidal volume before ligation.
    (1) greater than   (2) less than   (3) the same as

    b. The anatomic dead space would be ＿＿＿＿＿
    (1) increased.   (2) decreased.   (3) unchanged.

5. The important pressures influencing pulmonary blood flow are ＿＿＿＿＿＿＿

    a. alveolar.   b. pulmonary arterial.
    c. pulmonary venous.   d. none of these.
    e. all of these.

6. Compared with the blood coming to the lungs, the blood leaving them has ＿＿＿＿＿＿＿

    a. more carbon dioxide but less oxygen.
    b. more carbon dioxide and more oxygen.
    c. less carbon dioxide and less oxygen.
    d. less carbon dioxide and more oxygen.
    e. none of the above.

7. Assuming that $V_T = 600$ ml, $P_{E_{CO_2}} = 20$ torr, and $P_{A_{CO_2}} = 40$ torr,

    a. The respiratory dead space of a man breathing air is＿＿
    (1) 200 ml.   (2) 250 ml.   (3) 300 ml.
    (4) 350 ml.   (5) 400 ml.

    b. This suggests ＿＿＿＿＿＿＿
    (1) perfusion of poorly ventilated alveoli.
    (2) a low $\dot{V}/\dot{Q}$ ratio.
    (3) ventilation of poorly perfused alveoli.
    (4) true venous admixture.
    (5) a high $\dot{V}/\dot{Q}$ ratio.

8. a. Removing one lung from an individual would be expected to _____ the diffusing capacity as ordinarily measured.
       (1) increase   (2) decrease   (3) not affect

    b. The calculated carbon monoxide diffusing capacity while breathing CO in 40% oxygen would _____ compared with that while breathing CO in 29% O_2.
       (1) rise   (2) fall   (3) remain unchanged

Chapter 4

GAS TRANSPORT AND ACID-BASE BALANCE

As has been pointed out, the lungs act as the vehicle whereby oxygen is added to the blood and carbon dioxide is eliminated, while the tissues utilize oxygen and produce carbon dioxide. Clearly then, it is important to discuss the transport of these gases and their delivery to the lungs and the tissues, as well as the acid-base balance in the body.

OXYGEN IN THE BLOOD

The oxygen that diffuses from the alveoli into the pulmonary capillary blood is carried in the blood either as dissolved oxygen in physical solution in the plasma, or in combination with the hemoglobin in the erythrocytes.

The amount that dissolves in plasma is directly proportional to the partial pressure (.03 ml/torr/ℓ of plasma). Since the partial pressure of oxygen in the arterial blood in healthy individuals is approximately 100 torr, the amount of oxygen in physical solution in the plasma is about 3.0 ml/liter of plasma.

Most of the oxygen is carried in the erythrocytes in combination with hemoglobin as oxyhemoglobin. One gram of hemoglobin is capable of combining chemically with 1.34 ml of oxygen. In a healthy individual with a hemoglobin content of 15 g/100 ml, the blood is capable of carrying 20.10 ml of oxyhemoglobin per 100 ml of blood. The extent to which hemoglobin is actually combined with oxygen is usually expressed as the percentage saturation.

$$\text{saturation} = \frac{\text{oxygen content}}{\text{oxygen capacity}} \times 100$$

The saturation of hemoglobin depends upon the partial pressure of oxygen in the plasma, as is illustrated by the oxyhemoglobin dissociation curve (Fig. 4–1). The characteristic S-shape of this curve means that the hemoglobin clings to oxygen at the upper end of the scale, and gives up oxygen readily at lower oxygen tensions. The converse is also true, in that hemoglobin takes up oxygen very readily at lower oxygen tensions, but not at the upper end of the scale.

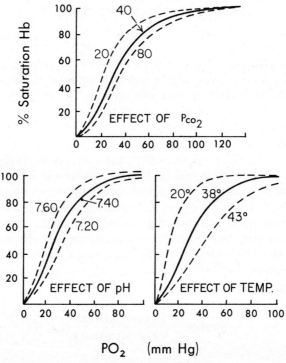

Figure 4–1. The graphs show the oxyhemoglobin dissociation curve (solid line) when the P_{CO_2} is 40 torr, pH is 7.40 and the temperature is 38° C. At low oxygen tensions, the hemoglobin takes up or gives up oxygen readily, while at high oxygen tensions the opposite is true. At a given partial pressure of oxygen, oxyhemoglobin will give up more oxygen when the carbon dioxide tension is higher, the pH is lower, or the temperature is elevated.

TISSUE OXYGEN

When the oxygenated blood reaches the tissues, oxygen diffuses rapidly from the blood into the tissue cells because the oxygen tension of the tissue cells is low (less than 10 torr). As a result, the partial pressure of the oxygen in the plasma falls. As we have seen from the oxyhemoglobin dissociation curve, hemoglobin relinquishes oxygen readily when the partial pressure of oxygen drops below 60 torr, so oxygen is liberated from the red blood cells into the plasma where it is then available to the tissues.

The amount of oxygen that will be given off to a particular tissue by the blood depends not only on the partial pressure of oxygen in that tissue but also on the partial pressure of carbon dioxide, the pH, and the temperature of the blood. Figure 4–1 demonstrates that, at a given partial pressure of oxygen, oxyhemoglobin will yield more oxygen when the carbon dioxide tension is increased, the pH lowered, or the temperature elevated. The effect of these variables is extremely important because they act as a safeguard for the welfare of the tissues. A fall in the partial pressure of oxygen in the tissue capillary blood, such as occurs when the activity of the tissues is increased or when the blood flow is decreased, is accompanied by a rise in carbon dioxide tension and hydrogen ion concentration. As a result, the dissociation curve is shifted to the right so that unloading of oxygen from the blood to the tissues is facilitated. Conversely, the fall in partial pressure of carbon dioxide tension as the blood passes through the lungs causes the dissociation curve to shift to the left, which increases the capability of hemoglobin to take on an additional quantity of oxygen.

CARBON DIOXIDE IN THE BLOOD

Several different chemical reactions play a role in the transport of carbon dioxide in the blood. The majority of the CO_2 that diffuses from the tissues into the systemic capillaries passes into the red cells, and is either carried as HCO_3^- or is bound to hemoglobin as carbamino compounds. Some of the carbon dioxide is also carried in the plasma, where it is present as HCO_3^-, or in simple solution in the plasma as dissolved CO_2. At normal body temperature, 0.067 vol per cent or 0.030 mM/ℓ of carbon dioxide will dissolve in the plasma for each torr of carbon dioxide. Since the arterial partial pressure of carbon dioxide in the arterial blood is normally about 40 torr, approximately 1.2 mM/ℓ of carbon dioxide is dissolved in the plasma. In the venous blood, where the carbon dioxide tension is approximately 46 torr, about 1.38 mM/ℓ of carbon dioxide is dissolved in the plasma.

Some of the dissolved carbon dioxide in the plasma reacts with water to produce carbonic acid (a process called hydration) which, in turn, dissociates into bicarbonate and hydrogen ions.

$$CO_2 + H_2O \rightleftarrows H_2CO_3 \rightleftarrows H^+ + HCO_3^-$$

Hydration of CO_2 in the plasma is a very slow chemical reaction, and the concentration of dissolved carbon dioxide is about 1000 times greater than the concentration of carbonic acid. Consequently only a small amount of bicarbonate is formed in the plasma. On the other hand, the hydration of carbon dioxide to carbonic acid is rapid in the red blood cells because they contain an enzyme called carbonic anhydrase, so that considerable bicarbonate is formed in the red cells.

The H^+ and HCO_3^- that result from the dissociation of H_2CO_3 in the red cells do not accumulate there. The hydrogen ions are mopped up by hemoglobin buffers, and some of the HCO_3^- moves into the plasma because the concentration in the red cells is much higher than it is in the plasma. The red blood cell membrane is relatively impermeable to cations, so the exit of the HCO_3^- anion creates an electrical imbalance. Electrical neutrality is preserved, however, because an equivalent amount of Cl^- ions move from the plasma into the red blood cells (a phenomenon called the "chloride shift").

In addition to carbon dioxide, which is a volatile acid, non-volatile acids such as H_2SO_4 and H_3PO_4 are generated by tissue metabolism. As we have seen, carbon dioxide is rapidly eliminated by the lungs, and normally the CO_2 equivalent of about 15,000 mEq of carbonic acid are eliminated by the lungs in a day. The dissociated hydrogen ions of the non-volatile acids are buffered and then slowly excreted by the kidney, only about 60 to 80 mEq of non-volatile (often called fixed) acids being excreted each day under normal circumstances. Clearly then, the respiratory system plays an important role in the regulation of the acid-base balance of the body. However, before discussing this role we must understand what is meant by many of the terms used in discussing acid-base relationships.

ACID-BASE BALANCE

ACIDS AND BASES

The terms **acid** and **base** are usually applied to proton (or hydrogen ion) donors or acceptors. It is customary to express the acidity or alkalinity of a solution by its pH, which is the negative logarithm to the base 10 of the hydrogen ion concentration. (This means that a decrease or increase of a pH unit represents a tenfold change in the opposite direction of the hydrogen ion concentration.)

Pure water, which is neutral, has a hydrogen ion concentration of about 10^{-7} moles/liter, so its pH is 7.0. By convention, a solution that has a hydrogen ion concentration greater than 10^{-7} moles/liter (i.e., pH < 7.0) is called an acid solution, and one that has a concentration lower than 10^{-7} moles/liter (i.e., pH > 7.0) is called an alkaline solution. As we will see, acidemia and alkalemia in the body denote very different levels of pH.

BUFFERS

The capacity of an acid-salt mixture to resist changes in pH is called its buffer action, and a mixture that can do this is called a buffer. The reaction of a solution that contains both acid and salt can be expressed by the equation

$$pH = pK + \log \frac{\text{buffer anion}}{\text{undissociated buffer}}$$

where pK is a constant that varies, depending on the types of acid and salt involved.

HENDERSON-HASSELBALCH EQUATION

The relationship between carbon dioxide (carbonic acid) and the anion bicarbonate in the plasma, which is reflected in the Henderson-Hasselbalch equation, is quantitatively the most important buffering system of extracellular fluid. The Henderson-Hasselbalch equation is used clinically to establish the existence and the severity of an acid-base disturbance

$$pH = pK + log \frac{HCO_3^-}{H_2CO_3}$$

where the pK for blood at body temperature is 6.10.

Since the concentration of H_2CO_3 is a thousand times less than that of dissolved carbon dioxide, which, in turn, is proportional to the partial pressure of CO_2, the equation may be rewritten

$$pH = 6.10 + log \frac{HCO_3^-}{0.0301 \times P_{CO_2}}$$

The balance between the bicarbonate and the dissolved carbon dioxide (or the carbon dioxide tension) is normally maintained at about 20:1 (Fig. 4–2). The bicarbonate level is normally about 24 mEq/ℓ and the dissolved carbon dioxide about 1.2 mEq/ℓ, and the pH is about 7.40 (range 7.35–7.45). Whenever this balance is disturbed secondary forces are called into play in an attempt to restore the balance and return the ratio of bicarbonate to dissolved carbon dioxide to about 20:1.

ABNORMALITIES OF ACID-BASE BALANCE

In discussing disturbances that result in abnormalities of acid-base balance, it is important to distinguish between the acid-base state of the blood and the abnormal

NORMAL ACID-BASE BALANCE

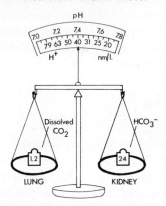

Figure 4–2. The balance between bicarbonate (24) and dissolved CO_2 (1.2 or $P_{a_{CO_2}} = 40$) is normally 20:1, and this is usually associated with a pH of about 7.40 and a H^+ concentration of about 40 mM/ℓ.

process that led to the primary disturbance. The abnormal acid-base states of the blood are **acidemia**, in which the hydrogen ion concentration (cH^+) is high and the pH low, and **alkalemia**, in which the cH^+ is low and the pH high. The abnormal processes leading to acid-base disturbances are **acidosis**, in which either a strong acid is gained or HCO_3^- is lost in excessive amounts, and **alkalosis**, in which either a strong base is gained or a strong acid is lost. The terms acidosis and alkalosis are further qualified according to the nature of the process that led to the primary disturbance.

A **respiratory acidosis** is an abnormal process in which the alveolar ventilation is not sufficient to cope with the rate of metabolic CO_2 production, so that **hypercapnia** is present. This is equivalent to the retention of the strong acid H_2CO_3. A **respiratory alkalosis** is an abnormal process in which the alveolar ventilation is excessive in relation to the metabolic CO_2 production, so that **hypocapnia** is present. This is equivalent to the loss of strong acid.

A **metabolic acidosis** is an abnormal process characterized by a primary gain of strong acid by the extracellular fluid (e.g., due to organic acids from metabolism, exogenous acids such as NH_4Cl, or a primary loss of HCO_3^- from the extracellular fluid through the kidney or the intestinal tract). A **metabolic alkalosis** is an abnormal process characterized by a primary gain of strong base by the extracellular fluid (e.g., due to the administration of exogenous HCO_3^-, or a primary loss of strong acid from extracellular fluid such as the loss of HCl from the stomach).

Thus we can see that the pH will be altered by pulmonary disturbances that cause changes in the carbon dioxide tension (i.e., the lung is underventilated or overventilated relative to the rate of carbon dioxide production), or by non-respiratory disturbances, more traditionally called metabolic disturbances, in which the rate of formation of hydrogen ions or their excretion by the kidney changes.

An acidosis will at first lead to acidemia, and an alkalosis to an alkalemia. However, if there has been compensation for the primary disturbance by a secondary process, then the hydrogen ion concentration in the blood may become normal. The degree of compensation may be complete or incomplete, and this is judged on the basis of whether or not the H^+ concentration or the pH has returned to a normal value. In the completely compensated state the primary disturbance (i.e., the acidosis or alkalosis) will still be present, but the acidemia or alkalemia will have been ameliorated. In simplified terms then, the pH can be looked upon as the balance between metabolic and respiratory functions.

$$pH = \frac{\text{metabolic (kidney)}}{\text{respiratory (lung)}} \quad \text{or} \quad \frac{HCO_3^-}{P_{CO_2}}$$

Respiratory Acid-Base Disturbances

A respiratory acid-base disturbance is present whenever the $P_{a_{CO_2}}$ deviates from the normal of 40 ± 5 torr. A $P_{a_{CO_2}}$ that is greater than 45 torr is called hypercapnia, or respiratory acidosis, and a $P_{a_{CO_2}}$ less than 35 torr is called hypocapnia, or respiratory alkalosis. As we have seen, the alveolar (and essentially the arterial) P_{CO_2} at any given point in time is dependent on the level of alveolar ventilation relative to the carbon dioxide production.

$$P_{CO_2} = \frac{\dot{V}_{CO_2}}{\dot{V}_A} \times 0.863$$

When a respiratory acid-base disturbance is the primary event, compensation is brought about by a physiologically induced metabolic disturbance (usually renal)—an alkalosis to correct a respiratory acidosis, and an acidosis to correct a respiratory alkalosis.

Respiratory Acidosis

When the alveolar ventilation is inadequate relative to the carbon dioxide production, the $P_{a_{CO_2}}$ rises (**respiratory acidosis**), so that the bicarbonate/dissolved carbon dioxide ratio becomes less than normal and, as a result, the hydrogen ion concentration rises (pH falls), i.e., **respiratory acidemia** is present (Fig. 4–3A). An acute reduction in total ventilation, or an increase in physiologic dead space but no compensatory increase in minute ventilation, without a proportionate reduction in carbon dioxide production will result in acute respiratory acido-

RESPIRATORY ACIDOSIS
AND ACIDEMIA

COMPENSATED RESPIRATORY
ACIDOSIS

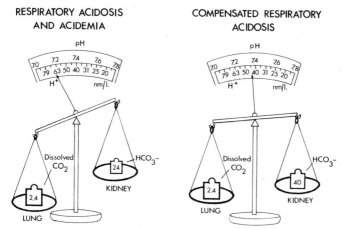

Figure 4–3. An elevated $P_{a_{CO_2}}$ means respiratory acidosis. In the acute situation the balance between HCO_3^- and dissolved CO_2 is less than 20:1, so that the pH is low (acidemia) and the H^+ concentration is elevated. With compensation by the kidney, bicarbonate is retained, so that the HCO_3^-/dissolved CO_2 ratio is closer to 20:1 and the pH and H^+ ion concentration are almost normal (but on the acidemic side).

sis and a resultant acidemia. A respiratory acidosis will also develop whenever the metabolic production of carbon dioxide rises without a proportionate increase in alveolar ventilation. This is particularly true when the work of breathing is excessive because, under such circumstances, any increase in ventilation may be associated with the production of more carbon dioxide than can be eliminated by the lungs.

When a respiratory acidosis and acidemia develop, the kidney increases the secretion of hydrogen ions, and reabsorbs and releases HCO_3 into the blood. There is an increased elimination of chloride in the form of HCl or NH_4Cl. The plasma Cl^- decreases by the same number of mEq/ℓ that the plasma HCO_3^- increases. This compensatory process begins immediately, but takes days to weeks to be maximal. If the renal compensation is complete, the bicarbonate/dissolved carbon dioxide ratio, and hence the pH, are restored to within the normal range (Fig. 4–3B).

Respiratory Alkalosis

When the alveolar ventilation is increased in relation to the CO_2 production, carbon dioxide is eliminated excessively, so that the $P_{a_{CO_2}}$ is low (**respiratory alkalosis**). Although the pH is protected to some extent by a reduction in the amount of reabsorption and generation of bicarbonate by the kidney, the bicarbonate/dissolved carbon dioxide ratio rises above 20:1. As a result the hydrogen ion concentration falls (pH rises), i.e., **respiratory alkalemia** is present (Fig. 4–4A). Respiratory alkalosis may develop because of direct or reflex stimulation of the central chemosensitive centers, due to a cerebrovascular accident or the ingestion of a drug that stimulates respiration (such as salicylate), or as a result of stimulation of the peripheral chemoreceptors by hypoxemia due to cardiorespiratory disease. It is also seen occasionally in highly emotional or apprehensive individuals.

When a respiratory alkalosis develops, the kidney begins to excrete more bicarbonate anions and excess cations while chloride ions are conserved. As a result the bicarbonate/dissolved carbon dioxide ratio is lowered toward normal and the pH tends to return toward the normal range (Fig. 4–4B). There is still controversy over whether the kidneys are capable of compensating completely for a chronic respiratory alkalosis, but it is generally thought that the compensation that takes place is

RESPIRATORY ALKALOSIS
AND ALKALEMIA

COMPENSATED RESPIRATORY
ALKALOSIS

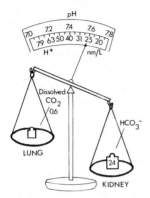
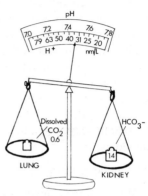

Figure 4–4. A reduced $P_{a_{CO_2}}$ means respiratory alkalosis. In the acute situation the balance between HCO_3^- and dissolved CO_2 is greater than 20:1 so that the pH is high (alkalemia) and the H^+ concentration is low. With compensation by the kidney, bicarbonate is excreted, so that the HCO_3^-/dissolved CO_2 ratio is closer to 20:1 and the pH and H^+ concentration are closer to normal (but on the alkalemic side).

incomplete, and that the pH remains above the normal range.

Metabolic Acid-Base Disturbances

At a given level of alveolar ventilation (or P_{CO_2}) the total number of positively charged cations (sodium, potassium, calcium, and magnesium) must equal the total number of negatively charged anions (chloride, bicarbonate, phosphate, sulfate, lactate, pyruvate, proteinate, and organic acids). The hydrogen ion concentration rises (i.e., pH falls) whenever their rate of formation is increased or their excretion through the kidney diminishes, or there is an increased loss of bicarbonate from the gastrointestinal tract because of diarrhea. The hydrogen ion concentration falls (i.e., pH rises) whenever there is an excessive loss of hydrogen ions from the stomach because of vomiting, or there is an accumulation of bicarbonate because of excessive ingestion.

When a metabolic disturbance is the primary event, compensation is brought about by a physiologically induced respiratory disturbance—an alkalosis to correct a metabolic acidosis, and an acidosis to correct a metabolic alkalosis.

Metabolic Acidosis

When there is an excess of hydrogen ions, as in diabetic ketosis, they react with bicarbonate to form carbonic acid. As Figure 4–5*A* demonstrates, the bicarbonate level falls (**metabolic acidosis**) and the bicarbonate/dissolved carbon dioxide ratio is reduced. There is a resultant increase in hydrogen ions, or a fall in pH (**metabolic acidemia**).

The increase in hydrogen ion concentration stimulates an increase in ventilation, so that more carbon dioxide is eliminated from the lungs and the $P_{a_{CO_2}}$ is secondarily lowered. In this way, the bicarbonate/dissolved carbon dioxide ratio tends to be returned toward normal, although it would appear that the respiratory response is never sufficient to completely restore the pH to normal (Fig. 4–5*B*).

Metabolic Alkalosis

When excess OH^- is present in the blood, it reacts with carbonic acid so that the bicarbonate level rises (**metabolic alkalosis**) and the bicarbonate/dissolved car-

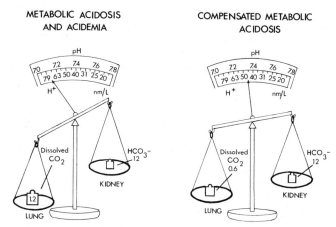

Figure 4–5. A reduced HCO_3^- means metabolic acidosis. In the acute situation the balance between HCO_3^- and dissolved CO_2 is less than 20:1 so that the pH is low (acidemia) and the H^+ concentration is high. With compensation by the respiratory system, CO_2 is eliminated so that the HCO_3^-/dissolved CO_2 ratio is closer to 20:1, and the pH and H^+ concentration are closer to normal (but on the acidemic side).

bon dioxide ratio is increased. As is illustrated in Figure 4–6*A*, there is a resultant reduction in hydrogen ions or a rise in pH (**metabolic alkalemia**). The concentration of chloride usually falls in association with the increase in bicarbonate.

As might be expected, compensation for a metabolic alkalosis is brought about by a reduction in ventilation due to inhibition of respiration by the reduced hydrogen ion concentration, so that the $P_{a_{CO_2}}$ rises (Fig. 4–6*B*). Under normal circumstances, however, the $P_{a_{CO_2}}$ does not rise above 50 torr, no matter how severe the metabolic alkalosis, so that compensation may not be complete.

From the foregoing it is clear that the respiratory sys-

METABOLIC ALKALOSIS   COMPENSATED METABOLIC
AND ALKALEMIA   ALKALOSIS

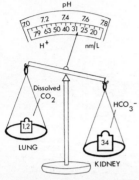 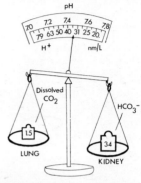

Figure 4–6. A raised HCO_3^- means metabolic alkalosis. In the acute situation the balance between HCO_3^- and dissolved CO_2 is greater than 20:1 so that the pH is high (alkalemia) and the H^+ concentration low. With compensation by the respiratory system, CO_2 is retained, so that the HCO_3^-/dissolved CO_2 ratio is closer to 20:1, and the pH and H^+ concentrations are closer to normal (but on the alkalemic side).

tem plays a major role in compensating for metabolic disturbances of acid-base balance. Because the neural mechanisms that influence the activity of the respiratory muscles (and hence the alveolar ventilation) are sensitive to changes in the acid-base state of the extracellular fluid, the $P_{a_{CO_2}}$ is altered so that the bicarbonate/dissolved carbon dioxide ratio (and therefore the pH) are restored to almost normal levels.

Mixed Acid-Base Disturbances

Pure acid-base disturbances such as we have discussed occur only briefly. Compensatory measures are introduced rapidly, and each of the four primary disturbances described is usually encountered with varying degrees of compensation. In addition, more than one disturbance of acid-base balance may occur at the same time, particularly in very ill people in whom there may be combinations of acute and chronic disorders. For instance, it is not uncommon to find that the pH is disproportionately low in patients with respiratory failure, particularly when shock or severe anemia is also present. Under these circumstances it may not be possible, on the basis of the blood data alone, to determine whether the hypercapnia is relatively acute and there has been little compensation, or whether hypercapnia has been present for some time and there has been compensation but an acute metabolic acidosis (such as a lactic acidosis) is superimposed on the underlying defect. Conversely, the pH may be found to be abnormally high in a patient with an elevated P_{CO_2}, i.e., a metabolic alkalosis exists along with the respiratory acidosis. Under these circumstances, the metabolic alkalosis may be the primary event and there has been respiratory compensation, or the respiratory acidosis may be the primary event and the concomitant metabolic alkalosis may have been induced by the administration of diuretic agents.

In general, in mixed disturbances the dominant disorder is usually reflected by the status of the pH. Nevertheless, in such circumstances, it is usually the clinical evaluation that serves as the only guide to the major disturbance.

SELF-ASSESSMENT

1. a. A low $P_{a_{CO_2}}$ may be found with _____
      (1) a metabolic acidosis.

     (2) a respiratory acidosis.
     (3) a metabolic alkalosis.
     (4) a respiratory alkalosis.
  b. A low arterial pH may be found with _____
     (1) a metabolic acidosis.
     (2) a respiratory acidosis.
     (3) a metabolic alkalosis.
     (4) a respiratory alkalosis.
  c. A high arterial total carbon dioxide content may be found with _____
     (1) a metabolic acidosis.
     (2) a respiratory acidosis.
     (3) a metabolic alkalosis.
     (4) a respiratory alkalosis.
  d. A high $P_{a_{CO_2}}$ may be found with _____
     (1) a metabolic acidosis.
     (2) a respiratory acidosis.
     (3) a metabolic alkalosis.
     (4) a respiratory alkalosis.
  e. A high arterial pH may be found with _____
     (1) a metabolic acidosis.
     (2) a respiratory acidosis.
     (3) a metabolic alkalosis.
     (4) a respiratory alkalosis.
  f. A low arterial total carbon dioxide content is found in _____
     (1) a respiratory acidosis.
     (2) a metabolic acidosis.
     (3) a metabolic alkalosis.
     (4) a respiratory alkalosis.
  g. A high plasma bicarbonate concentration may mean ____
     (1) a respiratory acidosis.
     (2) a respiratory alkalosis.
     (3) a metabolic alkalosis.
     (4) a metabolic acidosis.

2. In a metabolic acidosis
  a. The primary abnormality is reflected by ____ in HCO_3^-.
     (1) an increase   (2) a decrease   (3) no change
  b. and _____ in hydrogen ion concentration.
     (1) an increase   (2) a decrease   (3) no change

    c. This results in _____ in blood pH.
       (1) a rise   (2) a fall   (3) no change
    d. The change in blood pH will be ameliorated by _____
       (1) diminished alveolar ventilation
       (2) increased alveolar ventilation
       (3) increased urinary output
       (4) renal excretion of excess HCO_3^-
    e. and _____
       (1) a rise in P_{CO_2}.   (2) a fall in P_{CO_2}.
       (3) a fall in P_{O_2}.   (4) apnea.

3. Fill in the correct diagnosis.

	P_{CO_2}	pH	DIAGNOSIS
a.	25	7.25	_____
b.	65	7.36	_____
c.	40	7.55	_____
d.	70	7.55	_____
e.	25	7.50	_____

4. The arterial gases of a person with diabetic ketoacidosis are most likely to show _____
    a. $P_{CO_2} = 20$, pH = 7.55
    b. $P_{CO_2} = 20$, pH = 7.46
    c. $P_{CO_2} = 20$, pH = 7.30
    d. $P_{CO_2} = 50$, pH = 7.30
    e. $P_{CO_2} = 40$, pH = 7.40

5. The kidney and the lungs are the primary organs concerned with acid-base balance. Of those listed, the statement that best describes their regulatory function is _____
    a. The lungs can alter CO_2 very rapidly.
    b. The lungs usually respond to metabolic acidosis and acidemia by hyperventilating to produce a pH greater than 7.40.
    c. Renal compensation for respiratory acidosis is usually complete in 3 to 6 hours.
    d. All of the above.
    e. None of the above.

6. A patient's arterial pH is 7.55 and his arterial P_{CO_2} is 48

torr. These findings are consistent with a diagnosis of _____
a. voluntary hyperventilation.
b. acclimatization to high altitude.
c. asphyxia.
d. ingestion of excessive sodium bicarbonate.
e. severe renal insufficiency.

Chapter 5

CONTROL OF BREATHING

From the foregoing chapters it will be apparent that knowledge of the factors that influence breathing is essential. We have learned that alterations in respiration may interfere with gas exchange and acid-base balance, and that abnormalities of gas exchange may influence respiration, or that ventilation may be altered to compensate for acid-base disturbances. As the reader will realize, breathing can also be altered voluntarily by hyperventilating or breath-holding, and can be influenced by pain, apprehension, and excitement, all of which tend to augment respiration. The areas or "centers" that influence respiration are widely dispersed, and nerve cell collections that are involved in the regulation of breathing may be found in the cerebral cortex, hypothalamus, pons, and medulla, as well as the carotid and aortic bodies. These centers can be stimulated or inhibited by reflex action, or they can be affected directly by chemical stimuli. The neural control of respiration appears to play a minor role in the regulation of breathing in the human, when compared with the chemical control.

NEURAL CONTROL

Although reflexes such as the "Hering-Breuer reflex" or the "gasp reflex" have been shown to be active in animals and in newborn babies, their role in the control of breathing in adults is controversial. However, such reflexes may underlie the hyperpnea seen in patients who have developed an atelectasis or consolidation. Similarly, although mechanoreceptors in the airways give rise to hyperpnea and cough in response to irritants and may produce bronchoconstriction and systemic hypertension, their relative contribution to the tachypnea seen in pulmonary conditions is difficult to judge at the present time.

CHEMICAL CONTROL

Alterations of the carbon dioxide and oxygen tensions or hydrogen ion concentration in the blood exert a major influence on ventilation and have great clinical significance. Their effect on ventilation is mediated by chemosensitive areas in the ventrolateral surface of the medulla and peripheral chemoreceptors in the carotid and aortic bodies.

CARBON DIOXIDE STIMULATION

The most potent of all of the known chemical influences on ventilation is a rise in arterial carbon dioxide tension. If increasing percentages of carbon dioxide in air are inhaled, the ventilation increases in a relatively linear fashion and reaches a maximum of approximately 70 to 90 ℓ/min, when the concentration of carbon dioxide is 15 per cent. Stimulation of the chemosensitive areas in the medulla accounts for the majority of this increase in ventilation. Carbon dioxide can diffuse easily from the blood into these areas, but the blood-brain barrier does not allow hydrogen ions or bicarbonate to enter. Therefore when CO_2 diffuses into these areas, the local hydrogen ion concentration in the extracellular fluid will increase. It is generally believed that the chemosensitive areas are activated by the change in H^+ concentration in the extracellular fluid that is in direct contact with them. However, a rise in blood P_{CO_2} because of alveolar hypoventilation or the inhalation of carbon dioxide leads to dilation of the blood vessels in the brain, which in turn leads to an increase in the removal of carbon dioxide. The consequent lowering of the central P_{CO_2} tends to counteract the effect of hypoventilation on the composition of the extracellular fluid in the brain. Thus the ventilatory response to a change in arterial P_{CO_2} represents the integrated effect of several influences.

When the arterial P_{CO_2} is chronically elevated, as is the case in some patients with respiratory disease, the HCO_3^- concentration of the extracellular fluid in the central chemosensitive areas is also increased. As a result the local H^+ ion concentration is virtually normal. Under these circumstances, rapid lowering of the $P_{a_{CO_2}}$ by mechanical ventilation may induce deleterious effects.

Since carbon dioxide is freely diffusible across the blood-brain barrier, the P_{CO_2} in the central chemosensitive areas will also fall when the arterial P_{CO_2} is lowered. However, because the blood-brain barrier is impermeable to HCO_3^-, the HCO_3^- level in the chemosensitive areas will remain high. Consequently there will be an exaggerated fall in the hydrogen ion concentration in the chemosensitive areas, and this will depress ventilation. The alkalosis leads to cerebral vasoconstriction and, as a result, cerebral blood flow may be seriously impaired, and coma may ensue. Thus reduction of the $P_{a_{CO_2}}$ in patients with chronic hypercapnia should proceed slowly, so that there is sufficient time for the active processes that are involved in lowering the HCO_3^- concentration in the chemosensitive areas to become operative.

When the $P_{a_{CO_2}}$ falls below the normal range acutely, the opposite changes are seen. The low P_{CO_2} depresses ventilation and, if lowered considerably, may produce apnea. On the other hand, if a low carbon dioxide tension is maintained for a long period, as in a patient who is being artificially ventilated, spontaneous ventilation may be stimulated at even lower than normal levels of $P_{a_{CO_2}}$. The adaptation to a chronically low P_{CO_2} involves a reduction of the HCO_3^- concentration in the central chemosensitive areas, so that the hydrogen ion concentration in these areas is virtually normal. Consequently, a rise in P_{CO_2} will lead to an exaggerated increase in H^+ concentration when the HCO_3^- is low. Thus inhalation of CO_2 under these circumstances may actually lead to a greater ventilatory response than might normally be seen at the same P_{CO_2}. On the other hand, if hypocapnia has been induced artificially in a patient who is unable to ventilate adequately spontaneously, cessation of mechanical ventilation may result in the development of a severe acidemia.

HYPOXEMIC STIMULATION

A lower than normal $P_{a_{O_2}}$ normally leads to an increase in minute ventilation because hypoxemia stimulates collections of receptor cells in the carotid body and others that lie above and below the aortic arch. To a much lesser extent these receptors also respond to increases in $P_{a_{CO_2}}$ or H^+ concentration (fall in pH), a blood flow that is inadequate for their metabolic needs, or a rise in blood temperature. These stimuli may interact so that the degree of response to a given stimulus will depend on the coincident levels of other stimuli.

If an exceedingly brief period of hypoxemia is induced by the inhalation of a few breaths of a hypoxic gas mixture, ventilation will increase as soon as the oxygen tension falls below 90 mm Hg. On the other hand, during more prolonged inhalation of hypoxic gas mixtures, ventilation barely increases until the concentration of oxygen falls to about 14 per cent, which is equivalent to an altitude of 10,000 feet or a $P_{a_{O_2}}$ of approximately 60 torr. Even when the concentration of inhaled oxygen is reduced to 10 per cent and the $P_{a_{O_2}}$ is lowered to approximately 40 torr, the ventilation increases by only about 17 per cent. The maximal response, a ventilation of about 40 ℓ/min, occurs during the inhalation of 4 per cent oxygen in nitrogen, but hypoxemia of this severity can be tolerated for only a few minutes, and even then only at the risk of acute circulatory failure, unconsciousness, and convulsions.

The difference between the exceedingly brief and the more prolonged periods of exposure to hypoxic gas mixtures is probably explained by the compensatory mechanisms that take place in the latter situation. Indeed, if the exposure to the hypoxic gas were continued for a much longer period, the ventilation would increase further. These differing ventilatory responses to a hypoxemic stimulus are exemplified by the situation that one encounters on exposure to a higher altitude. Initially the fall in arterial oxygen tension will stimulate the carotid and aortic chemoreceptors and ventilation will be increased. As a result, the arterial (and brain) P_{CO_2} and hydrogen ion concentration will fall. This will inhibit the central chemosensitive areas and partially offset the stimulus resulting from impulses originating in the peripheral chemoreceptors. After a few days at that altitude the central hydrogen ion concentration will be restored to a normal level because the HCO_3^- level will fall. When fully adapted to altitude, both the blood and the central hydrogen ion concentration are normal, and under these circumstances the hyperpnea that results in response to the low P_{O_2} is unopposed by alkalemia in either the blood or the brain.

In healthy individuals the peripheral chemoreceptors do not play a major role in the control of breathing. However, in patients with chronic respiratory disease, hypoxemia may become an important stimulus to respiration. In such patients it has been suggested that chronic hypercapnia may lead to a reduction in the sensitivity of the medullary respiratory centers to P_{CO_2}, so that the peripheral chemoreceptors may become the principal regulators of the respiratory drive, and hypoxemia the primary stimulus to ventilation.

HYDROGEN ION STIMULATION

We have seen that the respiratory system brings about compensation for metabolic disturbances of acid-base balance by altering the level of ventilation. It is believed that metabolic acidemia and alkalemia respectively stimulate or depress ventilation over a range of arterial pH between 7.3 aand 7.5 through a direct effect on the peripheral chemoreceptors, whereas the central chemo-receptors are presumed to be affected when the pH is below 7.3 (and possibly also when it is above 7.5).

The adaptations to a metabolic acidosis or alkalosis are similar to those seen when there are changes in the P_{CO_2}. The hyperpnea that is induced by an acute meta-bolic acidemia causes the P_{CO_2} to fall in the arterial blood and the brain extracellular fluid. The resultant fall in hydrogen ion concentration in the brain reduces the central drive to ventilation and thereby offsets the full effect of the action of the peripheral chemoreceptors. After about 24 hours the hydrogen ion concentration in the brain becomes almost normal because of a propor-tionate reduction in HCO_3^-. Now the ventilation may be greater than normal because, under these circumstances, slight increases in P_{CO_2} are associated with greater than normal changes in hydrogen ion concentration. The sequence of events and the changes that develop are reversed when there is a metabolic alkalosis, such as occurs with excessive vomiting.

REGULATION OF VENTILATION IN RESPIRATORY DISEASE

In most patients with respiratory disease, minute ventilation is increased because of stimulation of either the central chemosensitive areas or the peripheral chemoreceptors. Aside from laboratory experimentation, it is unusual to find only a single chemical stimulus altered in patients with respiratory disease. Table 5–1 demonstrates that when ventilation is altered in response to a stimulus, other respiratory stimuli are also affected, and each makes a contribution to the total ventilatory response. For instance, in many patients with respiratory disease in whom hypoxemia is present because of mismatching of ventilation and perfusion, the ventilatory stimulation induced by the hypoxemia is to some extent counteracted by persistent hypocapnia as well as alkalemia.

In addition, it would appear that the activity of the respiratory centers may be modified when the work of breathing is high. Thus the minute ventilation falls even in healthy subjects when they breathe through an artificial airway obstruction. It appears that the body tolerates the resultant hypercapnia rather than expending the effort that would be required to lower the arterial P_{CO_2} and to keep it at a normal level. It has been suggested that the higher P_{CO_2} may actually be beneficial because any attempt to lower the $P_{a_{CO_2}}$ by increasing the ventilation might require so much oxygen that little would be available for non-ventilatory muscular work. In any case, these findings suggest that hypercapnia is

Table 5–1 THE ALTERATIONS IN CHEMICAL AGENTS DURING VARIOUS CONDITIONS

	ARTERIAL pH	ARTERIAL P_{CO_2}	ARTERIAL P_{O_2}
Inhalation of 5 per cent CO_2 in oxygen	↓	↑	↑
Inhalation of 10 per cent O_2 in nitrogen	↑	↓	↓
Voluntary hyperventilation	↑	↓	↑
Acute alveolar hypoventilation	↓	↑	↓

not as potent a stimulus to respiration when the work of breathing is increased.

As we learned in Chapter 2, the work of breathing may influence the respiratory pattern, the respiratory rate and depth being adjusted to the level at which the least amount of work or force will bring about the body's required alveolar ventilation. According to these considerations the respiratory frequency should increase when the elastic resistance is high (i.e., compliance is reduced) and decrease when the flow resistance is high. Indeed, the respiratory frequency increases (and the tidal volume falls) when normal subjects breathe against external elastic loading, and the frequency falls (and the tidal volume increases) with resistive loading. The respiratory patterns encountered in patients with respiratory disease often conform to these principles. This is particularly true in obese subjects or in patients with kyphoscoliosis in whom the compliance of the "chest wall" is low, or in pulmonary fibrosis when the compliance of the lungs is reduced. Here, as expected, the respiratory rate is high and the tidal volume low. In patients suffering from obstruction to airflow, on the other hand, respirations are also often rapid and shallow. This paradox has been attributed to the increase in end-expiratory level (FRC) in these conditions, which may also be an important determinant of the respiratory pattern.

SELF-ASSESSMENT

1. Ten minutes after a sudden ascent to an altitude of 20,000 feet

   a. ventilation is _____
      (1) increased.   (2) decreased.   (3) unchanged.

     b. arterial P_{CO_2} is _____
        (1) increased.   (2) decreased.   (3) unchanged.

     c. arterial pH is _____
        (1) increased.   (2) decreased.   (3) unchanged.

     d. arterial O_2 capacity is _____
        (1) increased.   (2) decreased.   (3) unchanged.

     e. arterial O_2 tension is _____
        (1) increased.   (2) decreased.   (3) unchanged.

     f. plasma HCO_3^- is _____
        (1) increased. (2) decreased. (3) essentially unchanged.

2. Indicate by arrows the acute deviation of change during the following conditions.

     ($\uparrow$ increase, $\downarrow$ decrease, $\leftrightarrow$ no change)

Condition	Alveolar Ventilation	P_{CO_2}	Arterial P_{O_2}	pH
a. Short duration inhalation of 5% CO_2 in 25% O_2 and 70% N_2				
b. Acute respiratory acidosis due to airway obstruction				
c. Inhalation of 10% O_2 in N_2 for a short duration				
d. Chronic metabolic acidosis without acidemia				
e. Voluntary hyperventilation				
f. Alveolocapillary block				

3. A man lived at 15,000 feet for two weeks. On his return to sea level he was found to have _____
     a. respiratory acidosis with acidemia.
     b. respiratory alkalosis with alkalemia.

    c. metabolic acidosis with acidemia.
    d. metabolic alkalosis with acidemia.

4. Chemoreceptor drive constitutes an important compensatory mechanism in _____
    a. carbon monoxide poisoning.
    b. anemia.
    c. methemoglobinemia.
    d. high altitude mountain climbing.

5. a. An acute increase in ventilation is noticed in most individuals when the O_2 content of the inspired air falls to
    (1) 20%.   (2) 15%.   (3) 10%.

   b. This increase is associated with _____ in CO_2 tension of the arterial blood.
    (1) a rise   (2) no change   (3) a fall

   c. The brain tissue P_{CO_2} _____
    (1) rises.   (2) falls.   (3) is unchanged.

   d. The brain hydrogen ion concentration _____
    (1) rises.   (2) falls.   (3) is unchanged.

SUGGESTED READING

Acid-Base Terminology. Report by Ad Hoc Committee of the New York Academy of Sciences Conference. Lancet, 2:1010, 1965.

Adams, W. R., and Veith, I.: Pulmonary Circulation. New York, Grune and Stratton, Inc., 1959.

Anthonisen, N. R., Danson, J., Robertson, P. C., and Ross, W. R. D. Airway closure as a function of age. Resp. Physiol., 8:58, 1969.

Anthonisen, N. R., and Milic-Emili, J.: Distribution of pulmonary perfusion in erect man. J. Appl. Physiol., 21:760, 1966.

Briscoe, W. A., and Dubois, A. B.: The relationship between airway resistance, airway conductance and lung volume in subjects of different age and body size. J. Clin. Invest., 37:1279, 1958.

Bryan, A. C., Bentivoglio, L. G., Beerel, F., McLeish, H., Zidulka, A., and Bates, D. V.: Factors affecting regional distribution of ventilation and perfusion in the lung. J. Appl. Physiol., 19:395, 1964.

Buist, A. S.: The Single Breath Nitrogen Test. New Eng. J. Med., 293:438, 1975.

Campbell, E. J. M., Agostoni, E., and Davis, J. N.: The Respiratory Muscles. Mechanics and Neural Control. Philadelphia, W. B. Saunders Co., 1970.

Cherniack, R. M., Cherniack, L., and Naimark, A.: Respiration in Health and Disease. Ed. 2. Philadelphia, W. B. Saunders Co., 1972.

Cherniack, R. M., and Snidal, D. P.: The effect of obstruction to breathing on the ventilatory response to CO_2. J. Clin. Invest., *35*:1286, 1956.

Comroe, J. H.: Physiology of Respiration. Ed. 2. Chicago, Year Book Medical Publishers, 1974.

Cumming, G.: Gas mixing efficiency in the human lung. Resp. Physiol., *2*:213, 1967.

Cunningham, D. J. C., and Lloyd, B. B. (Editors): The Regulation of Human Respiration. Proceedings of the H. S. Haldane Centenary Symposium, Oxford, 1961. Oxford, Blackwell Scientific Publications, 1963.

Davenport, H.: The ABC of Acid-Base Chemistry. Ed. 5. Chicago, University of Chicago Press, 1969.

Fenn, W. O.: Mechanics of respiration. Amer. J. Med., *10*:77, 1951.

Filley, G. F.: Acid-base and blood gas regulation. Philadelphia, Lea and Febiger, 1971.

Finch, C. A., and Lenfant, C.: Oxygen transport in man. New Eng. J. Med., *286*:407, 1972.

Finley, T. M., Swenson, E. W., and Comroe, J. H., Jr.: The cause of arterial hypoxemia at rest in patients with "alveolar-capillary block syndrome." J. Clin. Invest., *41*:618, 1962.

Forster, R. E.: Exchange of gases between alveolar air and pulmonary capillary blood. Pulmonary diffusing capacity. Physiol. Rev., *37*:391, 1957.

Fowler, W. S.: Intrapulmonary distribution of inspired gas. Physiol. Rev., *32*:1, 1952.

Hatcher, J. D., and Jennings, D. E. (Editors): Proceedings of the International Symposium on the Cardiovascular and Respiratory Effects of Hypoxia. New York, S. Karger, 1966.

Hills, A. G.: Acid-Base Balance. Chemistry, Physiology, Pathophysiology. Baltimore, The Williams and Wilkins Co., 1973.

Howell, J. B. L., and Campbell, E. J. M.: Breathlessness. Oxford, Blackwell Scientific Publications, 1966.

Hyatt, R. E.: The interrelationships of pressure, flow, and volume during various respiratory maneuvers in normal and emphysematous subjects. Amer. Rev. Resp. Dis., *83*:676, 1961.

Macklem, P. T.: Tests of lung mechanics. New Eng. J. Med., *293*:339, 1975.

Macklem, P. T.: Airway obstruction and collateral ventilation. Physiol. Rev., *51*: (No. 2). 368, 1971.

Macklem, P. T., and Mead, J.: Resistance of central and peripheral airways measured by a retrograde catheter. J. Appl. Physiol., *22*: 395, 1967.

McNeil, R., Rankin, J., and Forster, R. E.: The diffusing capacity of the pulmonary membrane and the pulmonary capillary blood volume in cardiopulmonary disease. Clin. Sci., *17*:465, 1958.

Mead, J.: Mechanical properties of the lungs. Physiol. Rev., *41*:281, 1961.

Milic-Emili, J.: Clinical methods for assessing the ventilatory response to carbon dioxide and hypoxia. New Eng. J. Med., *293*:864, 1975.

Milic-Emili, J., Henderson, J. A. M., Dolovich, M. B., Trop, D., and Kaneko, K.: Regional distribution of inspired gas in the lung. J. Appl. Physiol., *18*:749, 1966.

Milic-Emili, J., and Tyler, J. M.: Relation between work output of the respiratory muscles and end-tidal CO_2 tension. J. Appl. Physiol., *15*:377, 1960.

Otis, A. B.: The work of breathing. Physiol. Rev., *34*:449, 1954.

Otis, A. B., McKerrow, C. B., Bartlett, R. A., Mead, J., McIlroy, M. B., Selverstone, N. J., and Radford, E. P., Jr.: Mechanical factors in distribution of pulmonary ventilation. J. Appl. Physiol., *8*:427, 1956.

Schwartz, W. B., and Relman, A. S.: A critique of the parameters used in the evaluation of acid-base disorders. New Eng. J. Med., *268*: 1382, 1963.

Severinghaus, J. W., Bainton, C. R., and Carcelen, A.: Respiratory sensitivity to hypoxia in chronically hypoxic man. Resp. Physiol., *1*:308, 1966.

Siggaard-Andersen, O., and Engel, K.: A new acid-base nomogram. An improved method for the calculation of the relevant blood acid-base data. Scand. J. Clin. Lab. Invest., *12*:177, 1960.

Singer, R. B.: A new diagram for the visualization and interpretation of acid-base changes. Am. J. Med. Sci., *221*:199, 1951.

Weil, J. V., Byrne-Quinn, E., Sodal, I. E., Friesen, W. O., Underhill, B., Filley, G. F., and Grover, R. F.: Hypoxic ventilatory drive in normal man. J. Clin. Invest., *49*:1061, 1970.

West, J. B.: Respiratory Physiology; The Essentials. Baltimore, The Williams and Wilkins Co., 1974.

West, J. B.: Ventilation/Blood Flow and Gas Exchange. Oxford, Blackwell Scientific Publications, 1965.

West, J. B., Dollery, C. T., and Naimark, A.: Distribution of blood flow in isolated lung; relation to vascular and alveolar pressures. J. Appl. Physiol., *19*:713, 1964.

Whitelaw, W. A., Derenne, J. P., and Milic-Emili, J.: Occlusion pressure as a measure of respiratory center output in conscious man. Respir. Physiol., *23*:181, 1975.

Section II

ASSESSMENT AND INTERPRETATION OF PULMONARY FUNCTION

INTRODUCTION

There are a variety of tests that are used in order to detect whether there is a disturbance of respiratory function. These tests provide essential information about the impact of a disease on cardiopulmonary function, and are of particular benefit in assessing the extent of the disability present. They provide an objective evaluation of the progress of a disease process, and are of particular benefit to the physician in the evaluation of different modalities of therapy. Occasionally only one aspect of pulmonary function is altered by a particular disease and, in such cases, the studies may be very valuable in suggesting the correct diagnosis.

It is not the author's intention to discuss each individual technique in detail. Instead we shall discuss the general principles of methodology of some of the tests and the calculations that are carried out to determine the various parameters of function.

It is important to stress that *no* measurement or calculation is meaningful (and consequently no interpretation justified) unless the equipment that is used has been carefully calibrated, and the variability and reproducibility of the test validated in each particular laboratory. Quality control of the technician and the method of performing each test must be ensured. These requirements are applicable to even the simplest of tests, but are particularly true whenever electronic circuitry is involved. Again, it is not the intention to describe in detail the various steps that must be followed in order to ensure the accuracy of a particular piece of equipment that is being used to determine a parameter of respiratory function. Suffice it to say that any recording spirometer must measure volume and time accurately, a flow meter must measure flow rate accurately, and a gas analyzer must analyze gas concentrations accurately. For each apparatus that is used a calibration curve must be derived, and this curve must be checked at regular intervals to ensure that it is still applicable. When several sensing devices are used simultaneously in order to derive a particular parameter (such as thoracic gas volume or the mechanical properties of the lungs), one must ensure that the frequency response of the various instruments is adequate and that there is no phase lag between the electronic responses that will interfere with accurate measurement.

In this section we shall deal with spirometric tests of lung function including lung volumes, mechanics of breathing, and tests of ventilatory control, which are grouped under the headings of assessment of ventilatory function and tests of gas exchange.

Chapter 6

ASSESSMENT OF VENTILATORY FUNCTION

Tests that reflect the ventilatory function of the respiratory system may be altered by overall changes of either the elastic (i.e., compliance) or flow-resistive properties of the lungs and chest wall, or of the way that these properties vary throughout the lung. For instance, we have seen that the way gas is distributed in the lungs depends upon the distribution of regional time constants (i.e., the product of compliance and resistance). As we shall see, it is possible to measure the mechanical properties of the respiratory apparatus directly, but, in practice, simple spirometric tests that provide considerable insight into the status of the elastic and flow resistances are frequently used.

A valid interpretation of the measurements of mechanical properties of the lungs such as lung compliance or flow resistance (or even the simple spirometric tests) requires knowledge of the absolute lung volume at which these parameters were determined. Thus, wherever possible, the total lung capacity and its compartments should be determined when the forced vital capacity or the mechanical properties of the lungs are being assessed. The advent of the body plethysmograph has greatly improved our ability to assess the elastic or flow-resistive properties of the lung because lung volume can be de-determined at the same time, and any changes during the procedures can be monitored.

LUNG VOLUME

We have already learned that by using a simple spirometer we can determine the vital capacity (VC), the Expiratory Reserve Volume (ERV), and the Inspiratory Capacity (IC). However, to determine the absolute volume of gas in the lung and calculate the total lung capacity (TLC) one must know the residual volume (RV). This is usually derived by measuring the Functional Residual Capacity (FRC) and subtracting from it the ERV.

The FRC can be determined by utilizing either a dilution principle or a physical method that is based on Boyle's law. The techniques that utilize the dilution principle can be either single breath or multiple breath procedures in either a closed (rebreathing) or an open (non-rebreathing) system. The physical method, which employs a body plethysmograph to determine thoracic gas volume, is used most commonly nowadays. The physical method is quicker, is thought to be simpler, and is particularly useful because the flow resistance of the airways can be determined at the same time. On the other hand, the dilution techniques also provide a fringe benefit in that they provide additional information about the distribution of ventilation.

THE PHYSICAL METHOD
(BODY PLETHYSMOGRAPHY)

Boyle's law states that the volume of gas in a container varies inversely with the pressure to which it is subjected. This principle is applied in practice when the volume of gas in the lungs is determined in an airtight chamber (body plethysmograph). The thoracic gas volume is determined with the subject sitting in the body plethysmograph and breathing through a mouthpiece shutter system (Fig. 6–1). Since the air in the chamber heats up and is humidified by the subject's expirations, the pressure within the box rises rapidly after he first enters it. The pressure must be vented to the outside on repeated occasions until the pressure drift is minimal before measurements can be made. When there is little or no drift in the box pressure (indicating that the end-expiratory level is stable) the measurement of lung volume can be undertaken.

The principle behind the calculation of lung volume is simple: while the subject is breathing quietly through the mouthpiece, the gas in the subject's lungs is at at-

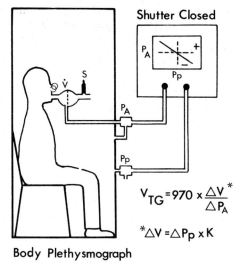

Shutter Closed

$$V_{TG} = 970 \times \frac{\Delta V}{\Delta P_A}^*$$

$$^*\Delta V = \Delta P_p \times K$$

Body Plethysmograph

Figure 6-1. This model illustrated the physical method of calculating lung volume (V_{TG}). The relationship (K) between volume change (ΔV) and pressure change in the box (ΔP_p) is determined so that pressure changes can be used to determine volume changes. When the shutter (S) is closed at FRC, the subject tries to inspire and expire so that the air in the chest is decompressed and compressed. As the chest volume increases the box volume decreases, and vice versa. The relationship between the mouth pressure (P_A) and the pressure in the box (P_p) is plotted on an oscilloscope. Since the pressure in the lungs at end-expiration was 970 cm H_2O, $V_{TG} = 970 \times \dfrac{\Delta P_p \times K}{\Delta P_A}$.

mospheric pressure at the points of end-inspiration and end-expiration where there is no airflow. If the shutter is closed at the end of a normal expiration, the gas within the chest will be trapped at that lung volume. The subject is then instructed to pant and make gentle inspiratory and expiratory efforts against the obstruction at a rate of approximately 120/min (while holding his hands against his cheeks to prevent gas movement into and out of the mouth). When this is done, the air in the chest will be alternately compressed and decompressed. During the compression and decompression, the relationship between changes in pressure measured at the mouth (which are equal to alveolar pressure) and changes in thoracic gas volume (as reflected by changes in pressure within the box) are observed continuously on an oscilloscope, the slope of this line being $\Delta P / \Delta V$. Unsatisfactory tracings will be obtained if the subject closes his glottis, or if the cheeks are allowed to balloon out or be sucked in during the breathing motions.

The pressure of the gas in the lungs at the onset of the test was 970 cm H_2O (atmospheric pressure minus water vapor pressure), and since the changes in pressure (ΔP) and volume (ΔV) during the panting procedure have been measured, it is possible to utilize Boyle's law to calculate the original volume of gas (V_{TG}) in the lungs.

$$P_I V_{TG} = (P_I + \Delta P)\ (V_{TG} + \Delta V)$$

where P_I is the initial pressure, $(P_I + \Delta P)$ the final pressure, and $(V_{TG} + \Delta V)$ the final volume.

then: $$P_I \Delta V + V_{TG} \Delta P + \Delta V \Delta P = 0$$

and $$V_{TG} = -\frac{\Delta V}{\Delta P}\ (P_I + \Delta P).$$

Since ΔP is very small compared to $(P_I + \Delta P)$, then as it approaches zero, $(P_I + \Delta P)$ approaches P_I and the equation becomes

$$V_{TG} = -P_I \times \frac{\Delta V}{\Delta P}$$

and if the sign is disregarded

$$V_{TG} = 970 \times \frac{\Delta V}{\Delta P}$$

Since the slope of the trace that we recorded on the oscilloscope was $\Delta P/\Delta V$, then the formula becomes

$$V_{TG} = \frac{970}{slope}$$

GAS DILUTION METHODS

Relatively insoluble gases such as helium or hydrogen (or the gas that is normally resident in the lung, i.e., nitrogen) are utilized in the gas dilution techniques. The system that is used can involve either multiple breath or single breath techniques.

Multiple Breath Helium Technique

In clinical laboratories where a body plethysmograph is not available, lung volume is often determined by a closed-circuit technique in which helium is utilized as the reference gas. In this test the subject inspires and expires from a spirometer containing 8 to 10 per cent helium in air and a carbon dioxide absorber. The test continues until equilibrium is reached (i.e., the concentration of helium is the same in the lungs and in the spirometer) and has remained stable for at least one minute. Sufficient oxygen (usually about 250 to 300 ml/min) is added to the system throughout the determination to keep the end-expiratory lung volume constant.

Knowing the volume of gas in the spirometer at the beginning of the test (V_S), the dead space of the spirometer and its tubing and the mouthpiece (V_{DS}), its helium concentration (F_I), and the helium concentration after equilibrium has been reached (F_E), one can calculate the volume of gas (V_{TG}) in the lungs from the following dilution equation

$$(V_{TG} + V_S + V_{DS})\, F_E = V_{TG}\,(F_O) + (V_S + V_{DS})\, F_I$$

Since the concentration of helium in the lungs at the beginning of the measurement (F_O) was zero, and if the initial inspiration from the spirometer began from the FRC, then

$$FRC = \frac{(V_S + V_{DS})\,(F_I - F_E)}{F_E}$$

Multiple Breath Nitrogen Clearance

In this method the nitrogen in the subject's lungs is washed out by successive inspirations of oxygen over a 7 minute period, while the expirations are collected in either a spirometer or a bag (open circuit). The subject is switched into a circuit that enables him to inspire 100 per cent oxygen at the end of a normal expiration.

From knowledge of the volume of oxygen breathed during the test, the amount of nitrogen that is washed out of the lungs, and the concentration of nitrogen left in the lungs at the end of the test, the volume of gas in the lungs at the onset of the measurement (FRC) can be derived

$$FRC = \frac{(V + V_{DS})(F_E - F_I)}{F_O - F_A} - C$$

where V is the volume of air expired; V_{DS} is the dead space of the spirometer, the tubing and mouthpiece; F is the concentration of N_2 in the expired gas (E), in the inspired oxygen (I), and in the alveoli at the onset of the test (O), and the end of the test (A). C is a correction factor for the N_2 excreted from the blood into the lung during the oxygen breathing.

Single Breath Helium Technique

The alveolar volume in the lungs can be determined from a single inhalation of a helium-air mixture. Usually it is calculated as a byproduct of the single breath estimation of the diffusing capacity using carbon monoxide (this technique will be described later). In this case, a vital capacity inspiration of the gas is carried out and the TLC is calculated

$$TLC \times F_E = (VC \times F_I) + (RV \times F_O)$$

Since the concentration of helium in the lungs at the onset of the inhalation (F_O) was zero, the equation for calculation of V_A (TLC) is

$$V_A = VC \text{ (BTPS)} \times \frac{F_I}{F_E}$$

where VC is the vital capacity inspired and F is the concentration of helium in the inspired (I) and the expired gas (E).

Single Breath Nitrogen Technique

In the single breath nitrogen test, a vital capacity inspiration of 100 per cent oxygen is followed by examination of the nitrogen in the vital capacity expirate. The residual volume is calculated from the dilution equation

$$(VC \times F_I) + (RV \times F_O) = TLC \times F_{\bar{E}}$$

where F is the concentration of N_2 in the inspired gas (I), in the lungs at the onset of inspiration (O), and in the mixed expired gas ($\bar{E}$).

The mixed expired or mean N_2 concentration ($F_{\bar{E}}$) is determined by collection of the total expirate in a container, or by planimetric or electrical integration of the moment-to-moment area under the expiratory N_2 concentration curve.

In this test RV is calculated. Since the concentration of nitrogen in the inspired gas (F_I) is zero (i.e., 100 per cent oxygen is inhaled) then

$$RV = VC \times \frac{F_{\bar{E}}}{F_O - F_{\bar{E}}}$$

CALCULATION OF TOTAL LUNG CAPACITY AND ITS SUBDIVISIONS

No matter which technique is used, the TLC and its subdivisions can now be determined with a simple spirometer. The calculations necessary depend on whether the thoracic gas volume was determined at the end of a normal expiration (i.e., at the resting level) so that the volume of gas determined is the FRC, or after a maximal expiration, where RV is the volume of gas determined, or at full inspiration, in which case the TLC is determined.

If the FRC has been determined then ERV and RV can be determined by having the subject expire maximally from FRC until no further air can be evacuated.

$$RV = FRC - ERV$$

And by having him inspire from the end-expiratory level until no further air can be inhaled, the IC and TLC can be determined

$$TLC = IC + FRC$$

If the volume that was measured was not FRC, the same manipulations can still be carried out and all the lung volume compartments determined. Since the FRC may vary with time, it is most appropriate to inspire to TLC whenever lung volume is being determined and then to calculate its subdivisions.

FORCED VITAL CAPACITY

One can derive considerable valuable information from a forced vital capacity maneuver, provided that the recording spirometer used has a very low flow resistance and a rapid response time.

The test consists of a forceful maximum expiration (FVC) beginning at full inspiration (TLC). The test may be performed with the subject in the sitting or standing position. No matter which position is utilized, the subject should be comfortable, and he should hold the tubing of the spirometer while his nose is occluded with a nose clip. The subject should be allowed to breathe normally until a constant end-tidal position is established over several consecutive breaths. Then he is instructed to inspire slowly as far as possible (to TLC), and then to blow out as hard and fast as possible (to RV). Since it is clear that this requires maximal cooperation, the technician must urge the subject on continuously ("keep blowing, keep blowing") until it is clear that no further air has come out of the lungs for several seconds. In most subjects the maneuver should last for at least 6 seconds. The procedure should be repeated at least 3 times until two reproducible maximal efforts are obtained.

The forced vital capacity (FVC) can be analyzed in several ways (Fig. 6–2). The absolute volume of the FVC is important in that it is an index of the state of the elastic properties of the respiratory system, whereas the rate at which it is expelled from the lungs is predominantly a reflection of the flow-resistive properties. Most laboratories assess flow resistance by an analysis of the volume of air expired in a particular time, the most frequent one being that expired in the first second ($FEV_{1.0}$). Some also measure the amount expired in the first half second ($FEV_{0.50}$) and in the first three quarters of a second ($FEV_{0.75}$).

Other commonly used analyses involve estimates of the rate of change of volume (i.e., the rate of airflow), the most frequent being the mean rate of airflow during the middle half of the forced expired vital capacity (the maximal mid-expiratory flow rate, or MMF). This is calculated by measuring the time taken for the middle 50 per cent of the vital capacity to be expired. The vital capacity is divided into 4 equal parts; the first 25 per cent

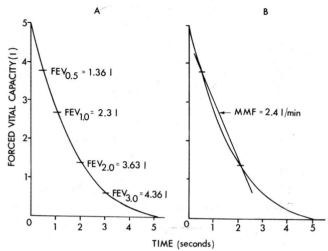

Figure 6–2. Flow resistance is assessed from the FVC in two ways: the volume of air expired in a particular period of time (A), such as 1/2, 1, 2, or 3 seconds; or the mean rate of air flow during the middle half of the FVC (B).

and last 25 per cent of the volume trace are ignored, and the middle 50 per cent of the vital capacity is divided by the time taken to expire it.

FLOW-VOLUME RELATIONSHIP

Currently many investigators examine the rate of air-flow as well as volume change during the forced expiratory maneuver, and they plot the relationship between the instantaneous expiratory flow rates (V_{max}) and volume throughout the forced vital capacity (Fig. 6–3), or report measurements of the airflow rate at particular lung

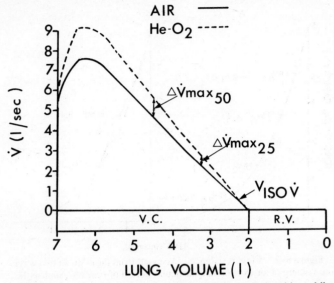

Figure 6–3. The graph shows the flow–volume relationships while breathing air and while breathing a helium-oxygen gas mixture. The two curves are superimposed on the absolute lung volume scale. Flow rates ($\dot{V}_{max}$) are higher when the helium-oxygen mixture has been breathed. The difference in $\dot{V}_{max}$ at 50% of the VC ($\Delta\dot{V}_{max}\,50$) and at 25% of the VC ($\Delta\dot{V}_{max}\,25$) as well as the volume at which flow rates become identical ($V_{iso}\dot{V}$) are usually reported.

volumes. If at all possible, the change in volume should be measured by a body plethysmograph because an artefact due to gas compressibility that is proportional to the subject's effort and the absolute gas volume will be present if volume is determined at the mouth. However, measurements of flow and volume at the mouth are also of value if expected "normal" values have been determined. Many laboratories report peak flow and the $\dot{V}_{max}$ after 25, 50 and 75 per cent of the vital capacity have been expired. It will be recalled that the maximal expiratory flow rates at high lung volumes (such as peak flow) are subject to wide variability and are very effort-dependent. Thus the flow rates after 50 ($\dot{V}_{max\ 50}$) and 75 ($\dot{V}_{max\ 25}$) per cent of the vital capacity have been expired are usually reported, because maximal effort is not necessary to produce a maximum flow over the lower two thirds of the lung volume.

HELIUM-AIR FLOW-VOLUME CURVES

Recently it has been suggested that the superimposition of flow-volume curves that are obtained during a forced expiration while the subject is inhaling a helium-oxygen mixture on that obtained while the subject is breathing air would provide a qualitative assessment of disturbance of "small airway" function. Thus, this test consists of the performance of a forced vital capacity maneuver while the subject is breathing air, and then again while he is breathing a helium (80%)- oxygen (20%) gas mixture. The two maximum flow-volume curves are superimposed, and the difference in flow rate at 50% of VC ($\Delta\dot{V}_{max\ 50}$) and at 25% of VC ($\Delta\dot{V}_{max\ 25}$) as well as the volume at which the two flow-volume curves intersect ($V_{iso}\dot{V}$) are then ascertained and reported (Fig. 6–3).

MAXIMUM BREATHING CAPACITY

The maximum breathing capacity (MBC), often also called maximum voluntary ventilation (MVV), is affected when the mechanical properties of the lungs and chest wall are altered, and is an index of the maximum ventilation achievable. In this test, which should be carried out with the subject in the standing position, the subject is instructed to breathe as deeply and as fast as possible for 12 to 15 seconds. The volume of air moved over this time period is extrapolated to 60 seconds, corrected to BTPS, and expressed in ℓ/min. This test is not used commonly any more. However, useful approximations of the MBC can be obtained from the product of $FEV_{1.0} \times 30$ or the $FEV_{0.75} \times 40$.

POST-BRONCHODILATOR STUDIES

Whenever the forced expiratory spirogram suggests that the flow resistance is greater than normal, the tests should be repeated following the inhalation of a nebulized bronchodilator.

In order to determine the effect of the bronchodilator, the method of administration of the aerosol is important. The subject should be asked to expire slowly, as far as possible (i.e., to RV), and then the nebulizer is placed in the subject's open mouth. The nebulizer bulb should be squeezed repeatedly (or the open limb of a Y-tube obstructed if a pressure source is being utilized) while the subject inhales very slowly, as if "sipping hot soup," to TLC. When full inspiration has been reached, the breath should be held for 2 to 3 seconds, and then expiration carried out slowly through pursed lips. This procedure should be repeated at 30 to 60 second intervals until the subject either "feels" the medication entering the lower lateral aspects of his chest, or the pulse increases, or jitteriness develops. When this occurs the subject should be allowed to rest for a few minutes, and then the spirometric tests should be repeated.

PULMONARY MECHANICS

As we learned in Chapter 2, it is possible to determine the mechanical properties of the respiratory system by simultaneous measurements of trans-pulmonary pressure, air flow and volume change. However, it is important to reiterate that calculation and interpretation of the interrelationship of the simultaneous electronic signals is only possible if their frequency responses are adequate and there is no phase difference between the balloon-catheter-transducer (pressure), pneumotachograph transducer (flow), and spirometer-transducer (volume) systems. Any phase lag must be corrected for, so that all of the systems are in phase.

ESOPHAGEAL PRESSURE

Although it is possible to obtain a direct measurement of the trans-pulmonary pressure in human subjects by inserting a needle into the pleural space through the chest wall, in practice the pressure in the esophagus is used because it records changes in intrapleural pressure quite faithfully. The esophageal pressure is sensed with a thin-walled balloon, usually about 10 cm long, that is attached to a 100 cm length of polyethylene tubing (number 200). The distal 9 cm of the polyethylene tubing (i.e., the part covered by the balloon) should have multiple holes in it.

The empty balloon should be inserted through the nose and swallowed into the stomach. About 1 ml of air should be injected into the catheter-balloon system, and then it should be connected to a pressure transducer.

Its presence in the stomach is confirmed if the pressure swings are positive on inspiration and negative on expiration. If this occurs, the balloon is retracted into the esophagus (this will be recognized by a change in the pressure swings—they will now be negative on inspiration and positive on expiration). The balloon should be retracted until it is about 10 cm above the point at which the pressure swings are noted to change. The exact position chosen should be the one at which the end-expiratory pressure is most negative and the effect of the heart beat the least (usually when the balloon tip is between 35 to 45 cm from the nares). The catheter should be fixed in this position by taping it to the nose.

To carry out any determinations of the mechanical properties of the lungs, the esophageal pressure measurements should be made with the balloon containing 0.5 ml of air. The volume of air in the balloon should be checked frequently when the mechanical properties of the lung are being studied. External leaks at the junctions of catheter to adaptors and other equipment will cause an increase in balloon volume, and a hole in the balloon will cause it to lose volume.

AIRFLOW AND VOLUME

Airflow is determined by means of a flow-measuring device (pneumotachograph) or by differentiating the volume signals from a spirometer. As was pointed out earlier, the ideal measurement of volume change in the chest is obtained by determining the pressure or volume changes in a body plethysmograph. Ordinarily volume is measured at the mouth, either with a spirometer, or by integration of the signal from a pneumotachograph.

Under these circumstances the volume must be corrected for changes in temperature or in the water vapor content of the gas. Throughout the studies of pulmonary mechanics, the points of zero airflow, pressure, and volume, as well as their calibrations, should be checked at repeated intervals.

ELASTIC PROPERTIES

Static Lung Compliance

To determine the elastic properties of the lungs, the relationship between the esophageal pressure and lung volume under static conditions is determined over the entire vital capacity range. The following procedure is usually followed: first, the subject is asked to inspire to TLC, and then to expire slowly to FRC. The pressure and volume are then measured while the mouthpiece is occluded for approximately 2-second intervals several times during a very slow inspiration from FRC to TLC, and a very slow expiration from TLC to RV. By plotting the absolute lung volume against the simultaneously recorded plateaus of trans-pulmonary pressure during the periods of interruption (zero airflow), a static pressure-volume curve of the lungs is obtained (See Figs. 2–6, 2–7, and 2–8). Since the static pressure-volume relationship is not linear and the lung compliance varies with the size of the individual (i.e., his lungs), the compliance is often calculated for a given volume change from FRC, and is then corrected for the lung volume at which it is measured; it is then called "specific compliance."

Dynamic Lung Compliance

When the compliance of the lungs is measured during breathing it is called the dynamic compliance. The volume change in a tidal breath is divided by the pressure change between end-expiration and end-inspiration (i.e., at points of zero airflow) as determined on the simultaneous record of airflow. If one measures the dynamic compliance at various respiratory frequencies (usually 20 to 60 breaths/min), one can determine whether the compliance is frequency-dependent. At least 10 breaths should be recorded.

The subject should be asked to inspire fully to TLC, and then expire to FRC, and then to breathe at a particular frequency (carried out in time with a metronome), within a predetermined tidal volume, keeping the end-expiratory volume constant. At least 10 breaths should be recorded at each frequency. After the subject has breathed the required number of breaths, he should immediately inspire to TLC. This allows calculation of the IC and ensures that there has been no drift in the volume signal.

The mean of the calculated dynamic compliance of each of the 10 breaths is calculated for each frequency, and is then usually expressed as a per cent of the static compliance that has been derived from the static pressure-volume relationship obtained during the slow inspiration from FRC to TLC.

Compliance of the Respiratory Apparatus

The compliance of the total respiratory apparatus (i.e., the lungs and chest wall) may be determined by measuring the pressure in the airway (at the mouth if the glottis is open) while the subject relaxes against a complete obstruction at the mouth at different lung volumes. As was discussed in Chapter 2 and illustrated in Figure 2–4, the plot of the relationship between these "relaxation" pressures and lung volume is called the **relaxation pressure curve**. The compliance of the total respiratory apparatus is calculated from the slope of this pressure-volume curve.

It is also possible to determine the compliance of the total respiratory apparatus by measuring the changes in the FRC, or resting level, that result when either a positive pressure is applied to the airway or a negative pressure is applied to the external surface of the chest.

Although it may seem that it is comparatively simple to determine the compliance of the total respiratory apparatus by utilizing these techniques, an accurate assessment can be obtained only when the respiratory muscles are either completely relaxed or even paralyzed. Complete relaxation of the respiratory muscles is extremely difficult to attain except in a well-trained subject, so this method is not always practical. Similarly, even though it is possible to determine the compliance when the respiratory muscles are paralyzed, one is never certain that the resistance to distention is similar to that present in the spontaneously breathing subject, in whom the compliance of the respiratory apparatus at FRC has been found to be approximately 0.12 ℓ/cm H_2O. From Figure 2–4 it is clear that if the static pressure-volume relationships of the lung are also determined, it is possible to calculate the compliance of the "chest wall." It will also be apparent that all estimates of compliance must be expressed in the light of the lung volume at which they are determined.

FLOW-RESISTIVE PROPERTIES

To determine the flow-resistive properties of the lung, one must obtain simultaneous measurements of airflow and the pressure required to overcome flow resistance. As we have already learned, the pressure required to overcome flow resistance is the sum of the pressures necessary to overcome the airway resistance, tissue viscous resistance, and inertia. The total flow resistance can be determined from simultaneous measurements of airflow, volume, and the esophageal pressure. However, in most laboratories the airway resistance is determined, since the tissue viscous resistance and inertia form only a small part of the total flow resistance.

Total Flow Resistance

It will be recalled that it is possible to separate the elastic and flow-resistive components of the trans-pulmonary pressure during a breath. This can be accomplished electronically during the determinations of pulmonary mechanics or from a plot of the relationship between the changes of volume and trans-pulmonary pressure during the breath (i.e., a pressure-volume loop). An example of a pressure-volume loop determined in a normal subject is illustrated in Figure 6–4. The elastic component of the trans-pulmonary pressure is derived by a line joining the points of zero airflow (end-expiration and end-inspiration) because the elastic resistance over the tidal volume range is linearly related to the state of lung distention. The pressure necessary to overcome flow resistance at any particular time is then determined by calculating the difference between the trans-pul-

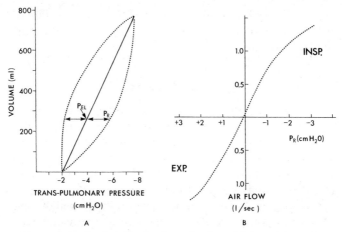

Figure 6–4. Depicted is the determination of flow resistance from the simultaneous relationship between volume and trans-pulmonary pressure (P_T) during a breath (A). The elastic component of the trans-pulmonary pressure (P_{EL}) is derived by a line joining the points of end expiration and end inspiration. The pressure necessary to overcome flow resistance (P_R) at any particular instant is the difference between P_T and P_{EL}. When P_R is plotted against the simultaneously measured rate of air flow (B), flow resistance can be derived from the slope of the linear portion of the curve ($\Delta P_R / \Delta \dot{V}$).

monary pressure and that required to overcome the elastic resistance at that instant

$$P_R = P_T - P_{EL}$$

Figure 6–4 also illustrates the relationship between the flow-resistive component of the pressure and the simultaneously measured rate of airflow (i.e., a pressure-flow plot). By convention, inspiration is usually plotted in the upper right quadrant and expiration in the lower left quadrant. Flow resistance is usually calculated by the slope of the pressure-flow plot over the linear portion of the curve, and is expressed as cm H_2O/ℓ/sec at a particular flow rate.

Airway Resistance

Two methods have been utilized to determine airway resistance. In one, the pressure at the mouth is determined during split second periods of obstruction to airflow at repeated intervals during the respiratory cycle. During the interruption of airflow, the pressure behind the obstruction is equal to alveolar pressure as long as the glottis is open. Although not always valid, one assumes that this pressure is the same as that which was present the instant before interruption, so that by relating the pressure to the flow rate just before the interruption, an estimate of airway resistance is obtained.

A much more common method of estimating alveolar pressure currently in use employs the body plethysmograph. In this case, the ratio between the changes in pressure at the airway opening (which are identical to alveolar pressure) and those in the body plethysmograph (which are opposite in sign) is determined (P_A/P_P) while the subject's airway is completely obstructed and the volume of air in the lungs is compressed and decompressed, just as in the determination of lung volume (Fig. 6–5). Then the relationship between the plethysmograph pressure and airflow while the subject pants (tidal volume of 100 to 200 ml at a rate of 120 to 200/min) through an unobstructed flow-meter is determined. The measurement is made during panting because this minimizes artefacts due to the warming and wetting of inspired air, the cooling and condensation of expired air, and the effect of the respiratory quotient.

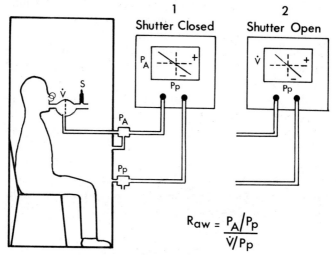

Body Plethysmograph

Figure 6–5. Measurement of airway resistance (R_{aw}) in the body plethysmograph is shown. With the shutter closed the ratio between mouth pressure (P_A) and box pressure (P_P) is determined. The relationship between P_p and airflow ($\dot{V}$)' is then estimated while the subject pants through the unobstructed pneumotachograph. Now $R_{aw} = P_A/\dot{V}$.

The slope of the relationship between the flow rate and plethysmograph pressure ($\dot{V}/P_P$) during the panting is measured between the points of inspiratory and expiratory flows of 1.0 ℓ/sec. Airway resistance is then calculated from the ratio of two slopes

$$R = \frac{P_A/P_P}{\dot{V}/P_P} \text{ in cm } H_2O/\ell/\text{sec}$$

The fact that this determination is made at the same time as lung volume is determined is particularly useful, since the airway resistance is dependent on the lung volume at which it is determined. Since the reciprocal of the flow resistance (**airway conductance**) is almost linearly related to lung volume, conductance per unit volume (**specific conductance**) is usually reported in most clinical laboratories.

Occasionally attempts are made to determine airway resistance during ordinary breathing. Under these circumstances one attempts to obviate as many of the artefacts as possible by having the subject breathe into and out of a rubber bag containing hot water that is located inside the chamber, so the temperature and saturation conditions of the respired air are constant throughout the respiratory cycle.

Upstream Resistance

As we have learned, only a small proportion of the flow resistance is present in the peripheral airways. Thus the measurements of airway resistance that have been described so far are not noticeably affected by alterations in the small peripheral airways. It is possible to measure the resistance in these peripheral airways because the lung elastic recoil is the driving pressure in the airways, which are upstream from the equal pressure point during a forced expiration.

Thus knowledge of the maximum expiratory flow rate ($\dot{V}_{max}$) achieved during a forced expiration at a particular lung volume and the elastic recoil pressure at that lung volume allows for the calculation of the flow resistance in these airways (R_{us})

$$R_{us} = \frac{P_{st}}{\dot{V}_{max}}$$

WORK OF BREATHING

Mechanical Work

As was pointed out earlier, the amount of mechanical work performed on the lung during breathing can be determined by deriving a pressure volume "loop" for each breath (Fig. 6–6). Estimation of the area contained within the trapezoid OABCDO yields the work performed to overcome the elastic resistance, while the area contained

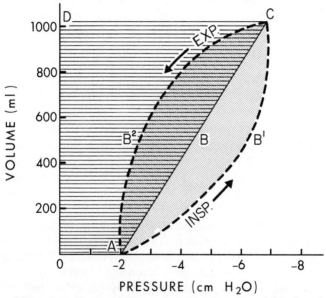

Figure 6–6. The graph shows the estimation of mechanical work performed on the lungs during a tidal breath. The cross-hatched area represents the work done to overcome elastic resistance, and the stippled area the work done to overcome flow resistance. Flow-resistive work during expiration is accomplished by the elastic recoil of the lungs.

within the loop $(AB'CB^2A)$ represents work performed to overcome flow resistance. Calculation of the area contained within the figure $OAB'CDO$ yields the total inspiratory work performed in that breath. If any of the loop falls outside of the zero pressure line, this must be added to the inspiratory work to determine the total work for that breath. If this calculation is representative of all breaths, it is multiplied by the respiratory rate to determine the work performed per minute.

Oxygen Cost of Breathing

The oxygen cost of breathing can be determined by means of either an open-circuit or a closed-circuit technique. In the open-circuit technique the subject either hyperventilates voluntarily at various levels of ventilation, or ventilation is measured while he inhales various concentrations of carbon dioxide. In the former case some CO_2 must be added to the inspired gas in order to prevent the development of hypocapnia. In both cases the expired air is collected after a steady state has been reached, and the expired gas concentrations are determined in order to calculate oxygen consumption.

In the closed-circuit technique the subject inspires and expires out of a spirometer containing 100% oxygen and a carbon dioxide absorber while breathing through varying lengths of dead space. After a steady state has been reached while breathing through a particular length of dead space, the minute ventilation and oxygen consumption (the slope of the end-expiratory points of the tidal volume excursions) are determined over a period of several minutes. The relationship between the minute ventilation and the oxygen consumption is then plotted to derive an oxygen cost curve (see Fig. 2–21).

DISTRIBUTION OF PULMONARY GAS

The overall manner in which gas is distributed in the lungs is influenced by the distribution of the mechanical properties of the lungs. The distribution of gas is assessed clinically with a foreign inert gas, as in determining lung volume, or a radioactive labeled gas. Both multiple breath and single breath methods employing closed-circuit or open-circuit techniques can be used.

Multiple Breath Helium Technique (Mixing Efficiency)

The rate at which the concentration of helium in a spirometer comes into equilibrium with that in a subject's lungs can be determined as a fringe benefit of the closed-circuit multiple breath helium technique used to determine lung volume. During the procedure the helium concentration is monitored continuously, along with tidal volume and respiratory rate, until the helium concentration plateaus, indicating that equilibrium has been reached.

To calculate the mixing efficiency, the number of breaths taken to reach 90 per cent of the equilibrium concentration is determined and compared with a calculated number of breaths that would theoretically be required to reach equilibrium in healthy lungs at FRC and with that particular tidal volume.

First the theoretical number of breaths is calculated. This requires knowledge of the tidal volume (V_T), the FRC, and the dead space of the apparatus (V_{DS})

$$\text{Theoretical number of breaths} = \frac{V_{DS} \times FRC}{V_T(FRC + V_{DS})}$$

$$\text{then: Mixing efficiency } (\%) = \frac{\text{Theoretical number of breaths}}{\text{Actual number of breaths}} \times 100$$

Nitrogen Washout (Multiple Breath Technique)

The manner in which oxygen is distributed in the lungs is determined during the multiple breath nitrogen techque for determining lung volume. The concentration of the expired N_2 at the mouth is monitored throughout the oxygen breathing, and the subject is asked to perform a maximal expiration at the end of the 7 minutes. The end-expiratory nitrogen concentration at the end of 7 minutes (i.e., the alveolar N_2 concentration) is called the "index of intrapulmonary mixing," and is less than 2.5 per cent in healthy individuals. A plot of the breath-by-breath nitrogen concentration over the entire 7 minute period allows for the derivation of "slow" and "fast" compartments in the lungs.

Single Breath Nitrogen Technique

Although single breaths of several foreign gases such as xenon[133], argon, or helium can be used to determine the manner in which gas is distributed in the lungs, it is the resident gas in the lungs, nitrogen, that is used as the marker gas in most clinical laboratories.

When a foreign gas is used, a bolus of the gas is inspired during the earliest part of a vital capacity inspiration from RV to TLC. When the resident gas technique is used, 100 per cent oxygen is inhaled throughout the vital capacity inspiration from RV. In both situations, this establishes a gas concentration difference between the alveoli at the top of the lung and those at the bottom at full inspiration. During the subsequent slow vital capacity expiration to RV, the concentration of the marker gas in the expirate and the change in volume are monitored continuously. Because considerable additional valuable information can be obtained from analysis of the plot obtained when nitrogen is the marker gas, the methodology of the single breath nitrogen technique will be described in detail.

The test is carried out while the subject is sitting. After breathing room air quietly for a few breaths, the subject is instructed to take two deep breaths and then exhale fully to RV. The subject is then switched to a pure oxygen source so that 100 per cent oxygen will be inhaled, and he is asked to inspire fully to TLC. Without breath-holding, the subject should then be asked to expire very slowly to RV (mean expiratory flow should be about 0.5 ℓ/sec and less than 0.7 ℓ/sec). The simultaneously recorded N_2 concentrations and volume changes during the ensuing full expiration should be displayed on an X-Y plotter or an oscilloscope. A minimum of 3 and a maximum of 6 such measurements are usually made, the number depending on the acceptance of the curves. An acceptable curve is one in which the inspired VC differs from the expired VC by less than 5 per cent and there is no step change in expired N_2 concentration in these curves. Ideally, the mean of 3, and at least 2, acceptable curves whose expiratory vital capacities are within 10 per cent of each other are reported.

A typical single breath N_2 curve is illustrated in Figure 6–7. As can be seen, the expired trace can be subdivided into several phases. Initially there is no nitrogen in the expired gas because it is gas from the anatomic dead space that has been filled with oxygen (Phase I). This is

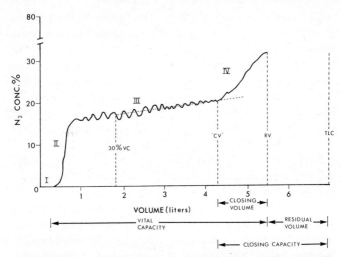

Figure 6–7. The Single Breath N_2 Curve. From this curve the anatomic dead space residual volume, total lung capacity, closing volume, closing capacity, and the slope of the alveolar plateau (Phase III) are frequently calculated.

followed by a phase in which alveolar gas mixes with gas from the dead space, and the curve has an S-shape (Phase II). From then on, the expired nitrogen concentration rises gradually (Phase III) until, at a low lung volume, there is an abrupt increase in the nitrogen concentration (Phase IV). From this trace a number of important parameters can be derived.

Anatomic Dead Space

Since the anatomic dead space (V_D) is full of oxygen at TLC, all the expired nitrogen must come from the alveoli. Thus calculation of the total amount of N_2 (V_{N_2}) that is expired in the vital capacity expiration allows for the calculation of the volume of gas that has been expired from the alveoli. Subtraction of this volume from the vital capacity yields the anatomic dead space

$$V_D = VC - (V_{N_2}/.7904)$$

Slope of Phase III

The slope of Phase III, an index of the uniformity of gas distribution, is determined by the best-fit line, which is drawn over the last half of the expired N_2 concentration/volume curve between the point at which 30 per cent of the VC has been expired and the onset of Phase IV.

Closing Volume

Closing volume (CV) is the component of the expiratory vital capacity that remains in the lung after the onset of Phase IV, i.e., the point of departure of the nitrogen concentration from a best-fit line that has been drawn through the latter half of Phase III. CV is usually expressed as a per cent of the expired vital capacity (CV/VC ratio).

Residual Volume

In relatively healthy individuals, residual volume (RV) can be calculated from the curve by the dilution equation, as was described earlier in this section.

Total Lung Capacity

As with other techniques, the total lung capacity (TLC) can be calculated by adding the vital capacity and the residual volume.

Closing Capacity

Closing capacity (CC) is the total volume of gas left in the lungs at the point of onset of Phase IV. Thus the closing capacity is composed of the closing volume and the residual volume (CV + RV), and is usually expressed as a per cent of total lung capacity (CC/TLC ratio).

Regional Distribution of Gas

In addition to the tests of overall gas distribution in the lungs, it is now possible to delineate the regional distribution of inspired gas by using a radioactive gas such as xenon[133] as the reference gas. Following the inhalation of the radioactive gas, the amount of radioactivity over different areas of the chest (often the upper, mid, and lower zones on both sides) is determined by means of counters placed over the chest or a scintillation camera while the subject holds his breath at full inspiration. The amount of radioactivity over these areas is also determined after the subject has rebreathed the radioactive gas from a spirometer until equilibrium has been reached, and then again holds his breath at full inspiration. This enables one to "calibrate" for different degrees of thickness of the chest wall and for regional lung volume, so that ventilation can be compared in different regions. Following the equilibration, it is possible to determine the rate of "washout" of radioactive gas from different regions of the lung by monitoring the changes in radioactivity during the subsequent expirations while the subject is inhaling room air.

CHEMICAL REGULATION OF VENTILATION

The respiratory response to chemical stimuli is assessed by measurement of the ventilation induced or the pressure developed by the inspiratory muscles against an occluded airway within 0.1 sec. ($P_{0.1}$) in response to changes in carbon dioxide or hypoxemia. The most recent advance in this area has revolved around the determination of occlusion pressure. Thus it is important to discuss the method of assessing occlusion pressure before discussing the various techniques of assessment of the chemical regulation of ventilation.

Occlusion Pressure

This measurement is made by having the subject breathe through a mouthpiece-valve arrangement that allows inspiration to take place through one tube and expiration through another. The inspiratory tube is obstructed during an expiration so that at the onset of the next inspiration, a negative pressure will be generated in the mouthpiece when the subject attempts to inspire. In practice, the pressure generated in the first 100 milliseconds ($P_{0.1}$) of the inspiratory effort is measured at irregular intervals throughout a study of the ventilatory response to CO_2 or hypoxemia. Because of the changing size of the respiratory system during breathing and differences in length (and therefore in the force that is developed) of inspiratory muscles, measurements of occlusion pressure must be made at a constant lung volume (i.e., at FRC). Since the end-expiratory lung volume does not appear to change perceptibly with increasing carbon dioxide when the subject is in the supine position, it has been recommended that this technique be utilized while the subject is in this position in order to study the output of the respiratory centers.

RESPONSE TO CARBON DIOXIDE

The response to carbon dioxide can be assessed utilizing either an open-circuit or a rebreathing technique. In

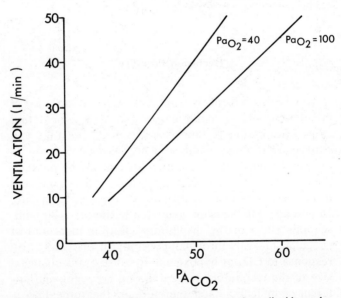

Figure 6–8. The ventilatory response to carbon dioxide under normoxic conditions ($P_{a_{O_2}} = 100$ torr) and hypoxemic conditions ($P_{a_{O_2}} = 40$ torr) is graphed. The slope of the relationship between $P_{A_{CO_2}}$ and ventilation while normoxic represents the response to CO_2. The difference between the ventilations at a particular $P_{A_{CO_2}}$ is indicative of the response to hypoxemia.

both cases, one plots the relationship between several levels of alveolar P_{CO_2} and the ventilation (Fig. 6–8) (or the $P_{.01}$) that has been induced, and then determines the slope of this relationship.

Steady State or Open-Circuit Technique

In the steady state or open-circuit technique, a gas containing carbon dioxide in air or in oxygen (so that any effect of hypoxemia is removed) is inhaled until a steady state is reached, or the minute ventilation is constant (usually 5 to 7 min). At this time, minute ventilation (and $P_{0.1}$) as well as the arterial or the end-tidal (alveolar) P_{CO_2} are recorded. Usually measurements of stimulus and response are made while the subject is inhaling carbon dioxide concentrations of 3, 5, and 7 per cent in oxygen.

Rebreathing or Closed-Circuit Technique

In this technique, the ventilatory response to carbon dioxide is determined while the subject is rebreathing from a small bag or a spirometer that at the onset of the measurement contains a volume of gas (6 to 7 per cent CO_2 in O_2) that is one liter greater than the subject's vital capacity. The end-tidal carbon dioxide tension and ventilation (tidal volume), which increase at a relatively constant rate with time, are measured continuously, while the $P_{0.1}$ is determined frequently at random intervals during the procedure. When average values for minute ventilation ($\dot{V}_E$) or the $P_{0.1}$ and the end-tidal carbon dioxide ($P_{A_{CO_2}}$) at 15 to 30 second intervals are plotted against each other, a linear relationship is usually obtained.

RESPONSE TO HYPOXEMIA

The response to hypoxemia is determined in virtually the same way as the response to carbon dioxide. In this case, however, it is essential to monitor the arterial gas tension changes because, as we have seen, the alveolar P_{O_2} and arterial P_{O_2} are not the same. In addition, the end-tidal carbon dioxide concentration must be kept constant at normocapnic levels during this test because the response will be enhanced if the P_{CO_2} is higher than normal, and inhibited if it is lower than normal.

Steady State or Open-Circuit Technique

In the steady state technique, gas mixtures containing oxygen concentrations between 12 and 20 per cent are inhaled. Under these circumstances carbon dioxide must be added to the inspired gas in order to keep the P_{CO_2} within the normal range. Otherwise the arterial P_{CO_2} will be lowered by the increased ventilation.

In another method of evaluating hypoxemic response, the ventilatory or $P_{0.1}$ response to inhaled carbon dioxide is determined while the alveolar or arterial P_{O_2} is maintained at normoxic levels (about 100 torr), and again when it is approximately 40 torr (Fig. 6–8). In this case, the difference in response at a particular P_{CO_2} is taken to represent the response to hypoxemia.

Rebreathing or Closed-Circuit Technique

The response to hypoxemia has also been determined by a re-breathing technique. In this case, air is rebreathed from a spirometer containing a carbon dioxide absorber, and sufficient CO_2 is added to the system to maintain a constant alveolar P_{CO_2}. The stimulus to breathing (hypoxemia) is monitored with an ear oximeter, which measures the oxygen saturation, and the response is determined on the spirometer, or by measuring $P_{0.1}$ at random intervals.

Chapter 7

ASSESSMENT OF GAS EXCHANGE

Tests of the gas exchange function of the lung are essentially performed to determine whether the blood leaving the lungs has approximately the same gas composition as the alveolar gas, and whether the values for arterial P_{O_2} and P_{CO_2} are normal. If they are not, the tests help to elucidate the mechanism of the abnormality.

We have seen that the exchange of gases in the lung takes place by the diffusion of gases between the alveolar ventilation and the pulmonary capillary blood, and that the distribution of the alveolar ventilation is influenced by the equality of the mechanical properties of the individual units within the lung. We have learned how to determine gas distribution, and so before discussing tests of gas exchange in the lung, it is essential to consider the other important element, the pulmonary blood flow.

PULMONARY BLOOD FLOW

As in the case of alveolar ventilation, it is possible to determine the absolute overall amount of pulmonary blood flow. Several techniques may be used.

The Fick principle can be utilized to determine the cardiac output or blood flow, and this entails knowledge of the oxygen consumption and the concentrations of oxygen in the arterial and mixed venous blood.

$$\text{Blood flow } (\ell/\text{min}) = \frac{\dot{V}_{O_2} \ (\text{ml/min})}{(a\text{-}\bar{v})_{O_2} \ \text{difference } (\text{ml}/\ell)}$$

Another method of determining the overall cardiac output or pulmonary blood flow involves the utilization of a dye dilution technique.

Pulmonary capillary blood flow can also be determined in a body plethysmograph, in which the volume changes are recorded as inhaled nitrous oxide gas is absorbed from the lungs into the blood stream. This technique is of special interest because it measures instantaneous flow through the pulmonary capillaries.

DISTRIBUTION OF BLOOD FLOW

Unlike the distribution of pulmonary gas, which can be assessed with simple inert gases, there is no simple technique for assessing the distribution of pulmonary blood flow that can be utilized by the majority of laboratories. Where this is required, radioactive gases or particles labeled with radioactive isotopes such as radioactive xenon[133] are utilized to determine blood flow distribution. The isotope is injected intravenously and, because of its low solubility, virtually all of it is evolved into the alveolar gas when it enters the pulmonary circulation and passes through the lung. By determining the amount of radioactivity over various regions of the chest using either counters or a scintillation camera (as was described earlier), its arrival in the lungs can be recognized. Then the amount of radioactivity present over the different regions is determined while the subject holds his breath at full inspiration in a manner similar to that described to determine the regional distribution of gas. As with the gas distribution study, the amount of radioactivity found over each chest region is corrected by the amount present when the lungs and spirometer were at equilibrium. In this way, the relative regional distribution of blood flow in the lungs can be described.

Macroaggregated albumin labeled with radioactive

iodine is also used to study the distribution of the pulmonary circulation, particularly when a pulmonary embolus is suspected. In this case, the intravenously injected albumin particles became lodged in small pulmonary vessels throughout the lung in a pattern determined by their blood flow, and this will be recognized by the relative amount of radioactivity present over the different parts of the lung fields. It must be pointed out that the distribution of these two isotopes is not necessarily the same. Thus the macroaggregated albumin displays the distribution of flow through all pulmonary vessels that are perfused, whereas the radioactive xenon technique demonstrates only blood flow through vessels that are going by alveoli that are ventilated.

DIFFUSION

Oxygen and carbon dioxide diffuse across the alveolocapillary membrane. In order to estimate the status of the diffusion characteristics of the lung, oxygen or carbon monoxide (which have a great affinity for hemoglobin) are utilized. The principles of the calculation of diffusing capacity are similar no matter which gas is being used.

DIFFUSING CAPACITY

In order to calculate the diffusing capacity, it is necessary to know the amount of the gas that is diffusing across the blood-gas barrier in a minute, and the mean difference in partial pressures of the gas between the alveolus and the pulmonary capillary.

Thus
$$D_{L_{O_2}} = \frac{\dot{V}_{O_2}}{P(\overline{A\text{-}c})_{O_2}}$$

and
$$D_{L_{CO}} = \frac{\dot{V}_{CO}}{P(\overline{A\text{-}c})_{CO}}$$

where D_L is the diffusing capacity of the lung in ml/torr/min, $\dot{V}$ is the volume of gas diffusing per minute, and $P(\overline{A\text{-}c})$ is the mean partial pressure gradient of the gas between the alveolus and the capillary.

We have seen that the amount of oxygen ($\dot{V}_{O_2}$) that diffuses across the blood-gas barrier in a minute (the oxygen uptake) is

$$\dot{V}_{O_2} = \dot{V}_E\,(F_{I_{O_2}} - F_{E_{O_2}})$$

Similarly, the amount of carbon monoxide ($\dot{V}_{CO}$) that is transferred across the blood-gas barrier in a minute is

$$\dot{V}_{CO} = \dot{V}_E\,(F_{I_{CO}} - F_{E_{CO}})$$

The mean difference in partial pressures of oxygen between the alveoli and the capillary is difficult to determine, since it varies along the course of the pulmonary capillary. The gradient is high at the point at which the venous blood arrives at the alveolus (about 60 torr), and is lowest at the end of the capillary where the partial pressures of the gas phase and the blood phase approach equilibrium (Fig. 7–1). For this reason, carbon monoxide is now used universally to assess the diffusing capacity of the lungs.

The mean gradient for carbon monoxide is much easier to estimate because it has a very high affinity for hemoglobin. Carbon monoxide can diffuse into the pulmonary

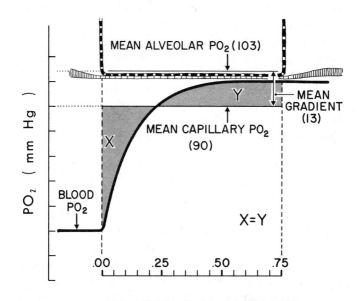

Figure 7–1. The oxygen tension varies along the course of the pulmonary capillary, and so does the alveolocapillary (A-c) gradient. The P_{O_2} in the mixed venous blood is about 40 torr, so that the A-c gradient is about 60 torr when the blood first enters the capillary. When the blood leaves the alveolus its P_{O_2} is virtually in equilibrium with that in the alveolus. The mean capillary P_{O_2} (X = Y) is about 90 torr, so that the mean A-c gradient is about 13 torr in this case.

capillary blood without producing a significant partial pressure in the plasma (i.e., the partial pressure of carbon monoxide in the pulmonary capillary blood is virtually zero). Thus, the mean alveolar carbon monoxide tension is considered equal to the gradient for carbon monoxide.

Both "single breath" and "multiple breath" "steady state" techniques of estimating the diffusing capacity of carbon monoxide ($D_{L_{CO}}$) are used. The single breath technique is easier to perform, but because the values are obtained under the artificial conditions of breathholding, they may not be as relevant to the "real life" situation as the "steady state" values.

Steady State Carbon Monoxide Diffusing Capacity

In this technique, the subject breathes a low concentration of carbon monoxide in air for several minutes, and the expired gas is collected in order to determine the amount of carbon monoxide transferred. The alveolar P_{CO} can be estimated in several ways. In one method the end-tidal CO concentration is monitored throughout the test, but this may be inaccurate when the tidal volume is small or if there is marked mismatching of ventilation and perfusion. In individuals with abnormal pulmonary function, therefore, alveolar carbon monoxide concentration is best obtained indirectly by calculating the physiologic dead space. If the dead space for carbon monoxide is the same as that for carbon dioxide, then

$$V_D = V_T \times \frac{P_{A_{CO_2}} - P_{E_{CO_2}}}{P_{A_{CO_2}}} = V_T \times \frac{P_{E_{CO}} - P_{A_{CO}}}{P_{I_{CO}} - P_{A_{CO}}}$$

and

$$P_{A_{CO}} = P_{I_{CO}} - \frac{P_{A_{CO_2}}}{P_{E_{CO_2}}} (P_{I_{CO}} - P_{E_{CO}})$$

Since the partial pressure of CO in the pulmonary capillary is virtually zero, then the alveolocapillary gradient is equivalent to the $P_{A_{CO}}$ and

$$D_{L_{CO}} = \frac{\dot{V}_{CO}}{P_{A_{CO}}}$$

Clearly the steady state technique depends on an accurate estimate of the mean concentration of carbon monoxide in the alveoli.

Single Breath Carbon Monoxide Diffusing Capacity

The single breath technique for estimating the $D_{L_{CO}}$ overcomes some of the difficulty of computing mean alveolar CO concentration.

In this test, the patient expires to RV and then inspires to TLC from a bag or spirometer containing a mixture of carbon monoxide and helium in air. The subject holds his breath for 10 seconds, and then expires fully to RV, the expired gas being collected in a bag.

To calculate the $D_{L_{CO}}$, the initial and final $F_{A_{CO}}$, alveolar volume, and the time from the onset of inspiration to the beginning of the alveolar sample collection must be determined.

The initial $F_{A_{CO}}$ is calculated from the $F_{I_{CO}}$ and the ratio of the expired to the inspired helium concentrations.

$$F_{A_{CO}} = F_{I_{CO}} \times \frac{F_{E_{He}}}{F_{I_{He}}}$$

The alveolar volume (i.e., TLC) is calculated from the

vital capacity and the ratio of expired to inspired helium concentrations.

$$V_A = \frac{VC(STPD)}{F_{E_{He}}/F_{I_{He}}}$$

then $\quad D_{L_{CO}} = \dfrac{V_A \times 60}{\text{Breath holding time (sec)} \times (P_B - 47)}$

$$\times \text{ Natural Log } \frac{F_{A_{CO}}}{F_{E_{CO}}}$$

The $D_{L_{CO}}$ is frequently corrected for the size of the lung and expressed as D_L/V_A ratio in ml/min/torr (STPD).

CARBON MONOXIDE EXTRACTION

Many clinical laboratories that determine $D_{L_{CO}}$ by the steady state technique also report the carbon monoxide extraction. This is the proportion of the inspired carbon monoxide that diffuses into the pulmonary capillary blood.

$$\% \text{ Extr.} = \frac{\dot{V}_E (F_{I_{CO}} - F_{E_{CO}})}{\dot{V}_I \times F_{I_{CO}}}$$

and since $\dot{V}_I = \dot{V}_E$, then

$$\% \text{ Extr.} = \frac{F_{I_{CO}} - F_{E_{CO}}}{F_{I_{CO}}}$$

PULMONARY CAPILLARY BLOOD VOLUME

The single breath $D_{L_{CO}}$ test is often varied in such a way as to obtain a measure of the diffusing capacity of the alveolocapillary membrane (D_M) as well as the pulmonary capillary blood volume. The principle behind these calculations is that the amount of CO taken up by the blood diminishes in the presence of increased oxygen levels because CO and O_2 compete for association with hemoglobin.

The resistance to diffusion of carbon monoxide ($I/D_{L_{CO}}$) is composed of the resistance offered by the blood gas barrier or membrane (M) and the chemical reactions in the blood (B)

$$I/D_{L_{CO}} = I/D_M + I/D_B$$

The blood term I/D_B is often expressed as the volume of CO that can be taken up by the blood in the pulmonary capillaries: i.e., $V_c \times \Theta$, where V_c is the volume of blood in the capillaries and Θ is the amount of CO that 1 ml of blood will take up for each torr partial pressure.

thus $$I/D_{L_{CO}} = I/D_M + I/V_c \times \Theta$$

The single breath $D_{L_{CO}}$ test is repeated on several occasions, utilizing a different concentration of oxygen each time. Then the reciprocal of each calculated $D_{L_{CO}}$ is plotted against the inspired oxygen concentration (Fig. 7–2). Analysis of the slope of this relationship provides an estimate of the volume of blood in the pulmonary capillaries (V_c), while the intercept on the scale repre-

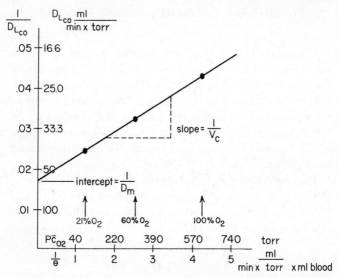

Figure 7–2. The $D_{L_{CO}}$ is measured on several occasions while the subject is breathing different concentrations of oxygen, in this case approximately 21% (air), 60%, and 100%. The pulmonary capillary blood volume (V_c) is represented by the slope of the relationship between the reciprocals of the $D_{L_{CO}}$ and the amount of CO taken up by 1 ml of blood at that particular partial pressure. The intercept of this slope represents the resistance of the membrane component (I/D_M).

senting $I/D_{L_{CO}}$ is indicative of the membrane component of the resistance to diffusion (I/D_M).

OVERALL ESTIMATION OF GAS EXCHANGE

In most clinical laboratories, an assessment of the adequacy of gas exchange is determined by the simultaneous collection of arterial blood and expired air while the subject is at rest and during exertion.

BLOOD AND GAS COLLECTION

The resting arterial blood and expired air are usually collected while the subject is semi-reclining. After the subject is in a steady state (RQ = 0.7 to .95), the expired gas is collected in a large spirometer or a collecting bag for a minute or longer, and the arterial blood is collected anaerobically over a number of breaths in the middle of the gas collection. In the majority of clinical situations, arterial blood is sampled on the clinical wards and expired gas is not collected. Once again however, the subject should be rested, and the blood drawn after the subject has been seated or in a semi-recumbent position for about 10 minutes.

Blood Sampling

Arterial blood samples are usually drawn from the radial or brachial arteries because they are the most accessible and safest sites of puncture. A 5 or 10 ml standard glass Luer-Lock syringe attached to a disposable 20 to 22 guage 1½ inch needle should be used. The syringe should be prepared by drawing sodium heparin into it and withdrawing and rotating the plunger several times so that the internal surfaces of the syringe and plunger are moist. Then all bubbles and the heparin should be expelled from the syringe while it is held in the upright position. This will leave about 0.2 ml of heparin in the dead space of the syringe and needle, which is adequate for anticoagulation.

The skin over the area chosen for puncture should be cleansed with an alcohol swab, and the needle then directed into the artery at about a 45° angle. Entry of the needle into the artery will be recognized by pulsation of blood into the syringe. It is not necessary to pull on the plunger if the needle is in an artery because the blood pressure itself will force blood into the syringe unless the patient is in shock. When the desired amount of blood is in the syringe, the needle should be withdrawn from the artery and inserted into a rubber stopper. If there are any bubbles in the blood they should be expelled immediately while the syringe is held in the upright position.

After withdrawing the needle, firm pressure must be applied to the puncture site for at least 5 minutes. This is extremely important, since delayed bleeding into the tissues, which can be very painful, is common.

Gas Analysis

Analyses of the gas tensions and pH should be performed immediately on the freshly drawn blood sample. If the analyses cannot be carried out immediately, the sample should be stored anaerobically in ice water in order to minimize changes due to the metabolic activity of the blood cells.

The analysis of arterial P_{O_2}, P_{CO_2} and pH is carried out with blood electrodes and, in some laboratories, the oxygen and carbon dioxide content of the blood are also measured. The gas concentrations in the expired air can be measured by the same electrodes or with gas analyzers. Clearly any blood or gas sample must be introduced into the electrodes without exposure to ambient air because both the P_{O_2} and P_{CO_2} as well as pH of the blood will change if it is exposed to any bubbles of air.

The electrodes must be carefully thermostated in order to maintain a constant temperature within $\pm 0.1°$ C of the body temperature of $37°$ C at all times. For routine laboratory determinations all parameters of blood gases should be assessed at a constant temperature of $37°$ C. When the patient's temperature is different, the measured P_{O_2} must be corrected to obtain the value that actually existed at the patient's temperature.

The Oxygen Electrode

The oxygen electrode is essentially a silver anode and a platinum wire (cathode) that is immersed in a dilute solution containing reducible or oxidizable substances. When the electrode is placed in such a solution containing O_2 and a suitable voltage is applied to it, the oxygen is reduced and electrons will pass from the cathode to the anode. This transfer of electrons is measured by a galvanometer, the amount of current flowing being proportional to the number of oxygen molecules present, i.e., to the partial pressure of oxygen in a gas. When this electrode is used to determine the oxygen tension in blood, it is covered with a polyethylene membrane that is permeable to gases.

The pH Electrode

The apparatus used to measure the pH consists of an electrode made of a thin glass membrane, which is freely permeable only to H^+ ions, plus a reference electrode (Ag/AgCl), both of which are in a reference solution of saturated KCl. The latter is in electrolytic connection with the saturated solution of KCl, and the KCl, in turn, has a liquid junction with the sample being measured. An electrometer that is connected to the reference electrode and a calomel electrode measures the electrical potential generated by the transfer of hydrogen ions across the glass membrane between the sample being measured and the reference solution.

The CO_2 Electrode

The Severinghaus CO_2 electrode is also a special glass electrode that is permeable to H^+. It is surrounded by a thin film of bicarbonate-containing electrolyte, which is separated from a blood or gas sample by a thin Teflon membrane that is permeable to gases but not to hydrogen ions. When a sample of gas or fluid containing CO_2 is exposed to the membrane, the molecules of CO_2 diffuse through the Teflon membrane and react with the water in the electrolyte solution to form H^+ and HCO_3^- ions. The H^+ ions, in turn, pass through the glass electrode where $Ag/Ag\,Cl$ electrodes measure their concentration, as in a pH meter.

Indirect Measurement of $P_{a_{CO_2}}$

When an arterial puncture is difficult or undesirable, it is still possible to obtain a reliable estimate of arterial P_{CO_2} by monitoring the CO_2 concentration at the mouth while the subject rebreathes from a bag that was initially filled with oxygen and a small amount of CO_2. During rebreathing the CO_2 concentration will plateau when the carbon dioxide in the lung-bag system is equal to the mixed venous P_{CO_2} ($P_{\bar{v}_{CO_2}}$). Unless the cardiac output is abnormal, the arterial P_{CO_2} at rest can then be estimated by assuming that the arteriovenous P_{CO_2} difference is about 6 torr.

CALCULATION OF PARAMETERS OF GAS EXCHANGE

Once the gas concentrations in the expired air and the partial pressures of oxygen and carbon dioxide in the arterial blood have been measured, it is possible to calculate many parameters that are of considerable value in the interpretation of respiratory disturbances. The parameters that are usually determined are the oxygen consumption ($\dot{V}_{O_2}$), carbon dioxide production ($\dot{V}_{CO_2}$) and respiratory quotient (R), the physiologic dead space (V_D) and dead space-tidal volume ratio (V_D/V_T), and the effective alveolar partial pressure of oxygen ($P_{A_{O_2}}$); this in turn allows for the derivation of the alveolo-arterial O_2 partial pressure difference or gradient ($P(A-a)_{O_2}$), and the amount of venous admixture.

Oxygen Consumption

As we have already seen on several occasions, the oxygen uptake or consumption per minute ($\dot{V}_{O_2}$) is determined by calculating the difference between the amount of oxygen that is inhaled and the amount exhaled.

$$\dot{V}_{O_2} = (\dot{V}_I \times F_{I_{O_2}}) - (\dot{V}_E \times F_{E_{O_2}})$$

where $\dot{V}$ is the ventilation/minute and F the concentration of oxygen in the inspired (I) and the expired (E) air. And since the amount of air inspired/minute is equal to that expired, one usually collects and measures the volume of air expired/minute

$$\dot{V}_{O_2} = \dot{V}_E \times (F_{I_{O_2}} - F_{E_{O_2}})$$

The oxygen consumption is conventionally expressed at STPD.

Carbon Dioxide Production

Like the oxygen consumption, carbon dioxide production ($\dot{V}_{CO_2}$) is determined from the difference between the amount exhaled and that inhaled, and is expressed at STPD.

$$\dot{V}_{CO_2} = \dot{V}_E \times (F_{E_{CO_2}} - F_{I_{CO_2}})$$

Since there is virtually no carbon dioxide in the ambient air (0.04%), the $\dot{V}_{CO_2}$ is determined by collecting the expired air and measuring its CO_2 concentration.

$$\dot{V}_{CO_2} = \dot{V}_E \times (F_{E_{CO_2}} - 0.04)$$

Respiratory Quotient

The respiratory quotient or ventilatory gas exchange ratio (R), is represented by the ratio of the $\dot{V}_{O_2}$ and $\dot{V}_{CO_2}$.

$$R = \frac{\dot{V}_{CO_2}}{\dot{V}_{O_2}} = \frac{\dot{V}_E (F_{E_{CO_2}} - F_{I_{CO_2}})}{\dot{V}_E (F_{I_{O_2}} - F_{E_{O_2}})}$$

and

$$R = \frac{F_{E_{CO_2}} - F_{I_{CO_2}}}{F_{I_{O_2}} - F_{E_{O_2}}}$$

Physiologic Dead Space

The physiologic dead space (V_D) is that portion of the tidal volume that does not take part in gaseous exchange. It is usually calculated from the Bohr equation, using carbon dioxide as the reference gas. This is based on an analysis of the source of the carbon dioxide in an expired breath (V_T).

$$V_T \times F_{E_{CO_2}} = (V_A \times F_{A_{CO_2}}) + (V_D \times F_{D_{CO_2}})$$

Since $V_A = V_T - V_D$, and the concentration of CO_2 in the dead space is the same as that of the inspired air (i.e., virtually zero), the equation becomes

$$V_T \times F_{E_{CO_2}} = (V_T - V_D) \times F_{A_{CO_2}}$$

and

$$V_D = V_T \times \frac{F_{A_{CO_2}} - F_{E_{CO_2}}}{F_{A_{CO_2}}}$$

or when expressed in terms of the partial pressures

$$V_D = V_T \times \frac{P_{A_{CO_2}} - P_{E_{CO_2}}}{P_{A_{CO_2}}}$$

while the dead space/tidal volume ratio is

$$V_D/V_T = \frac{P_{A_{CO_2}} - P_{E_{CO_2}}}{P_{A_{CO_2}}}$$

As long as the lungs are healthy, the end-tidal P_{CO_2} is a fairly accurate reflection of the mean $P_{A_{CO_2}}$. However, in patients with cardiorespiratory disease it is difficult to

obtain a representative alveolar sample, so that in practice arterial P_{CO_2} is used instead of alveolar P_{CO_2} to calculate the physiologic dead space.

"Ideal" Alveolar P_{O_2}

The status of the arterial oxygen and carbon dioxide
tensions and the alveoloarterial P_{O_2} difference tell us
about the adequacy of gas exchange.

Unlike the arterial P_{O_2}, which we can measure directly,
the true alveolar P_{O_2} cannot be measured. Instead we
calculate an "ideal" or "effective" value for alveolar P_{O_2}
utilizing $P_{a_{CO_2}}$ and the alveolar air equation. This is based
on the assumption that the arterial P_{CO_2} is representative
of the mean P_{CO_2} in the perfused alveoli, and that the gas
exchange ratio of these alveoli is equal to that of the
lungs as a whole.

$$P_{A_{O_2}} \text{ (ideal)} = F_{I_{O_2}}(P_B - 47) - P_{A_{CO_2}}\left(F_{I_{O_2}} + \frac{I - F_{I_{O_2}}}{R}\right)$$

Although this equation looks formidable, in fact it is
quite simple to estimate the ideal $P_{A_{O_2}}$. The first part of
the equation is simply the partial pressure of moist inspired air. The latter part in brackets will vary with the
inspired oxygen concentration and the respiratory quo-
tient. Finally, $P_{a_{CO_2}}$ is used instead of $P_{A_{CO_2}}$. If 100 per
cent oxygen is inhaled, the value within the brackets
becomes I, and the equation is simply the difference between the inspired P_{O_2} and the $P_{A_{CO_2}}$.

$$P_{A_{O_2}} = P_{I_{O_2}} - P_{a_{CO_2}}$$

As we have pointed out earlier, in the majority of

clinical situations the expired gas is not collected along with the arterial blood sample, so the respiratory quotient cannot be calculated. However, if room air were being breathed while the blood was drawn, a respiratory quotient of 0.8 is assumed; $P_{a_{CO_2}}$ is substituted for $P_{A_{CO_2}}$ and a simplified verision of the equation is used.

$$P_{A_{O_2}} = P_{I_{O_2}} - \frac{P_{a_{CO_2}}}{0.8}$$

or

$$P_{A_{O_2}} = P_{I_{O_2}} - (P_{a_{CO_2}} \times 1.25)$$

Alveolo-Arterial P_{O_2} Difference or Gradient

The effective alveolar oxygen tension is used to determine the gradient or difference between the mean alveolar and the arterial oxygen tensions $(P(A-a)_{O_2})$. In normal persons the A-a gradient varies between 5 and 15 torr while room air is being inhaled, depending on the age of the individual.

Venous Admixture

The calculated $P_{A_{O_2}}$ can also be utilized to determine the amount of venous admixture present, i.e., the proportion of the cardiac output that is acting like a shunt. These calculations are based on equations that utilize either the arterial oxygen content or saturation.

$$\frac{\dot{Q}_s}{\dot{Q}_T} = \frac{C(c' - a)_{O_2}}{C(c' - \bar{v})_{O_2}}$$

or

$$\frac{\dot{Q}_s}{\dot{Q}_T} = \frac{S(c' - a)_{O_2}}{S(c' - \bar{v})_{O_2}}$$

where C is the content and S the saturation of oxygen in the end-capillary (c'), arterial (a), and mixed venous ($\bar{v}$) blood. It is usually assumed that the mean $P_{c'_{O_2}}$ is the same as the effective $P_{A_{O_2}}$, and the end-capillary and arterial oxygen contents and saturations are estimated from the respective oxygen tensions. The mixed venous content is usually estimated by assuming an a-$\bar{v}$ difference, and in most circumstances an a-$\bar{v}$ content difference of 5 vol per cent and a saturation difference of 25 per cent are assumed.

In practice, this approach is frequently utilized to derive a qualitative estimate of the amount of true right to left shunt. The test essentially consists of the determination of the arterial P_{O_2} after the subject has been breathing 100 per cent oxygen for 20 minutes. If the hemoglobin in the pulmonary end-capillary and the arterial blood is fully saturated (this is a perfectly valid assumption if the P_{O_2} is greater than 100 torr), a difference in oxygen content between the end-capillary and arterial blood resulting from a greater than normal amount of shunting of poorly oxygenated blood into oxygenated blood will be reflected in the oxygen that is in physical solution in the blood.

For instance, if, while breathing 100 per cent oxygen, the $P_{a_{O_2}}$ is 500 torr and $P_{a_{CO_2}}$ is 40 torr in a person whose hemoglobin is 20 gm/100 ml, the $C_{a_{O_2}} = 20.0 \times 1.34$ (O_2 carried by hemoglobin) + $500 \times .003$ (O_2 in solution) = 28.30 ml/100 ml of blood.

since $\quad P_{A_{O_2}} = P_{C'_{O_2}}$

then

$$P_{c'_{O_2}} = 760 \ (P_B) - 47 - 40 \ (P_{a_{CO_2}}) = 673 \ torr$$

and

$$C_{c'_{O_2}} = (20 \times 1.34) + (673 \times .003)$$
$$= 28.82 \text{ ml/100 ml of blood}$$

If the a-$\bar{v}$ oxygen content difference is 5 ml/100 ml, then

$$\frac{\dot{Q}_s}{\dot{Q}_T} (\% \text{ shunt}) = \frac{28.82 - 28.30}{28.82 - 23.30} \times 100 = 9.4\%$$

ACID-BASE BALANCE

The current availability of relatively simple equipment for measurement of pH and P_{CO_2} has facilitated the study of acid-base balance to the extent that it is an essential part of the assessment of any patient with metabolic or respiratory disturbances. As was described earlier, the sample of arterial blood must be obtained anaerobically if the status of the acid-base balance in the body is to be determined. Measurement of any two of the three variables of the Henderson-Hasselbalch equation (i.e., pH, P_{CO_2} and CO_2 content) allows for the calculation of the third variable.

CALCULATION OF ACID-BASE STATUS

The approach to the measurement of parameters necessary to characterize the acid-base status varies in different laboratories. In most laboratories, the P_{CO_2} and pH are both measured with electrodes, and the total CO_2 content and bicarbonate concentration are calculated. In others, the pH of blood and the total CO_2 content of whole blood or plasma (with a Van Slyke apparatus) are determined, and the P_{CO_2} and bicarbonate ion concentration are calculated from the Henderson-Hasselbalch equation. Some laboratories also express the acid-base state of the patient in terms of blood buffer base (which is the sum of the conjugate bases, and includes bicarbonate and non-bicarbonate buffers) and in terms of "standard bicarbonate" (which is the bicarbonate concentration of the blood sample when it is equilibrated with a gas with a P_{CO_2} of 40 torr). The term "base excess" is used to describe the amount in mEq/liter by which the observed value for buffer base exceeds the expected value, whereas "base deficit" is used to describe the amount by which it is lower than the expected normal. The determination of the expected whole blood buffer base and the extent of base excess and base deficit are derived from nomograms.

EXERCISE TESTS

The assessment of gas exchange during exercise is especially important in the evaluation of pulmonary function because an abnormality may only become evident during exercise. Although not always possible, the level of exercise chosen for assessment of exercise performance in patients should be close to one that is limited by symptoms. Clearly this means that the patient must be closely observed during the exercise test, so that it can be halted immediately should untoward signs appear.

The technique of Jones and Campbell for evaluating the response to exercise on a cycle ergometer or treadmill is most useful and informative. In this technique, the exercise workload is increased progressively at minute intervals, by equal increments (about 100 Kilipound meters or about 17 watts/min in adults), until the heart rate exceeds 130/min. The approximate equivalent measures of exercise intensity are shown in Table 7–1.

Table 7–1   MEASURES OF EXERCISE INTENSITY

CYCLE ERGOMETER (Kpm/min)	POWER OUTPUT WATTS	OXYGEN INTAKE (ℓ/min)	ENERGY EXPENDITURE (kcal/min)	EVERYDAY ACTIVITY
300	50	1.0	5	Walking 3 mph
600	100	1.5	7.5	Walking 4.5 mph
900	150	2.0	10	Running 6 mph

In addition to the subject response, the cardiac frequency (EKG), blood pressure, ventilation, tidal volume, and frequency of breathing should be determined at each exercise load. In addition, if facilities are available, oxygen uptake and carbon dioxide output should be measured. Should the response to exercise be abnormal, a more detailed assessment is carried out at two or three of the workloads, and these are chosen on the basis of the initial tests. At each workload, measurements should be made after the cardiorespiratory variables have reached a steady state (usually 3 to 5 minutes). In addition to the measurements mentioned above, the concentration of gases in the expired air and the mixed venous carbon dioxide tension (using the rebreathing technique) should be determined and arterial blood (or arterialized blood) sampled.

With these measurements, it is then possible to determine the dead space/tidal volume ratio and the

$P(A-a)_{O_2}$. In addition it is possible to determine the cardiac output. An empirical correction is applied to the oxygenated $P_{\bar{v}CO_2}$ that is obtained by rebreathing, and the $C_{\bar{v}CO_2}$ is derived from the CO_2 dissociation curve. Then, knowing the $\dot{V}_{O_2}$, $\dot{V}_{CO_2}$, and the $P_{\bar{v}CO_2}$, the a-$\bar{v}$ oxygen content difference $C(a-\bar{v})_{O_2}$ and the cardiac output can be estimated from the nomograms derived by McHardy et al.

SUGGESTED READING

Bates, D. V., Woolf, C. E., and Paul, G. I.: Chronic bronchitis. A report on the first two stages of the coordinated study of chronic bronchitis in the Dept. of Veterans Affairs, Canada. Med. Serv. J. Canada, *18*:211, 1962.

Boren, H. G., Kory, R. C., and Syner, J. C.: The Veterans Administration-Army cooperative study of pulmonary function II. The lung volume and its subdivisions in normal men. Am. J. Med., *41*:96, 1966.

Buist, A. S.: The single-breath nitrogen test. New Eng. J. Med., *293*: 438, 1975.

Burrows, B., Knudson, R. J., and Kettel, J.: Respiratory Insufficiency. Chicago, Year Book Medical Publishers Incorporated, 1975.

Despas, P. F., Leroux, M., and Macklem, P. T.: Site of airway obstruction in asthma as determined by measuring maximal expiratory flow breathing air and a helium-oxygen mixture. J. Clin. Invest., *51*:3235, 1972.

Dickman, M. L., Schmidt, C. D., and Gardner, R. M.: Spirometric standard for normal children and adolescents (ages 5 years through 18 years). Am. Rev. Respir. Dis., *104*:680, 1971.

Dosman, J., Bode, F., Urbanetti, J., Martin, R., and Macklem, P. T.: The use of a helium-oxygen mixture during maximum expiratory flow to demonstrate obstruction of small airways in smokers. J. Clin. Invest., *55*:1090, 1975.

DuBois, A. B., Botelho, S. Y., Bedell, G. N., Marshall, R., and Comroe, J. H., Jr.: A rapid plethysmographic method for measuring thoracic gas volume: a comparison with a nitrogen washout method for measuring functional residual capacity in normal subjects. J. Clin. Invest, *35*:322, 1956.

DuBois, A. B., Botelho, S. Y., and Comroe, J. H., Jr.: A new method for measuring airway resistance in man using a body plethysmograph: values in normal subjects and in patients with respiratory disease. J. Clin. Invest., *35*:327, 1956.

Frohlich, E. D.: Pathophysiology: Altered Regulatory Mechanisms in Disease. Ed. 2., Philadelphia, J. B. Lippincott Co., 1976.

Hackney, J. D., Sears, C. H., and Collier, C. R.: Estimation of arterial CO_2 tension by rebreathing technique. J. Appl. Physiol., 12:425, 1958.

Jones, N. L.: Exercise testing in pulmonary evaluation. Rationale, methods and the normal respiratory response to exercise. New Eng. J. Med., 293:541, 1975.

Jones, N. L.: Exercise testing in pulmonary evaluation: clinical applications. New Eng. J. Med., 293:647, 1975.

Jones, N. L.: Exercise testing. Brit. J. Dis. Chest, 61:169, 1967.

Jones, N. L., Campbell, E. J. M., Edwards, R. H. T., and Robertson, D.: Clinical Exercise Testing. Philadelphia, W. B. Saunders Co., 1975.

Jones, N. L., Campbell, E. J. M., McHardy, G. J. R., Higgs, B. E., and Clode, M.: The estimation of carbon dioxide pressure of mixed venous blood during exercise. Clin. Sci., 32:311, 1967.

Kory, R. C., Callahan, R., Boren, H. G., and Syner, J. C.: The Veterans Administration Army cooperative study of pulmonary function. I. Clinical spirometry in normal men. Am. J. Med., 30:243, 1961.

Lindal, A., Medina, A., and Grismer, J. T.: A re-evaluation of normal pulmonary function measurements in the adult female. Am. Rev. Resp. Dis., 95:1061, 1967.

Leuallen, E. C., and Fowler, W. S.: Maximum mid-expiratory flow. Am. Rev. Tuber., 72:783, 1955.

Macklem, P. T.: Tests of lung mechanics. New Eng. J. Med., 293:339, 1975.

McHardy, G. J. R.: Relationship between the difference in pressure and content of carbon dioxide in arterial and venous blood. Clin. Sci., 32:299, 1967.

McHardy, G. J. R., Jones, N. L., and Campbell, E. J. M.: Graphical analysis of CO_2 transport. Clin. Sci., 32:289, 1967.

Milic-Emili, J.: Clinical methods for assessing the ventilatory response to carbon dioxide and hypoxia. New Eng. J. Med., 293:864, 1975.

Miller, W. F., Johnson, R. L., Jr., and Wu, N.: Relationships between fast vital capacity and various timed expiratory capacities. J. Appl. Physiol., 14:157, 1959.

Polgar, G., and Promadhat, V.: Pulmonary Function Testing in Children: Techniques and Standards. Philadelphia, W. B. Saunders Co., 1971.

Read, D. J. C.: A clinical method for assessing the ventilatory response to carbon dioxide. Australas. Ann. Med., 16:20, 1967.

Rebuck, A. S., and Campbell, E. J. M.: A clinical method for assessing the ventilatory response to hypoxia. Am. Rev. Respir. Dis., 109:345, 1974.

Schilder, D. P., Roberts, A., and Fry, D. L.: Effect of gas density and viscosity on the maximal expiratory flow-volume relationship. J. Clin. Invest., *42*:1705, 1963.

Schmidt, C. D., Dickman, M. L., Gardner, R. M., and Brough, F. K.: Spirometric standards for healthy elderly men and women. Am. Rev. Respir. Dis., *108*:933, 1973.

Severinghaus, J. W.: Electrodes for blood and gas pCO_2, pO_2 and blood pH. Acta Anaesthesiol. Scand. (Suppl.), *11*:207, 1962.

Sinclair, M. J., Hart, R. A., Pope, H. M., and Campbell, E. J. M.: The use of Henderson-Hasselbalch equation in routine medical practice. Clin. Chem. Acta, *19*:63, 1968.

Stein, M., Tanabe, G., Rege, V., and Khan, M.: Evaluation of spirometric methods used to assess abnormalities in airway resistance. Am. Rev. Resp. Dis., *93*:257, 1966.

United States Department of Health, Education and Welfare, National Heart, Lung and Blood Institute, Division of Lung Diseases: Suggested standards for closing volume determination (Nitrogen Method), 1973.

Weil, J. V., Byrne-Quinn, E., Sodal, I. E., Friesen, W. O., Underhill, B., Filley, G. F., and Grover, R. F.: Hypoxic ventilatory drive in normal man. J. Clin. Invest., *49*:1061, 1970.

Whitelaw, W. A., Derenne, J. P., and Milic-Emili, J.: Occlusion pressure as a measure of respiratory center output in conscious man. Respir. Physiol., *23*:181, 1975.

Wood, L. D. H., and Bryan, A. C.: Effect of increased ambient pressure on flow-volume curve of the lung. J. Appl. Physiol., *27*:4, 1969.

Chapter 8

INTERPRETATION OF PULMONARY FUNCTION

We now know that the assessment of pulmonary function is an essential component of the clinical evaluation of all patients with respiratory complaints. Pulmonary function tests provide information about the mechanism of disturbance present. In most cases the tests of function help the physician to determine the amount of disability present, and to follow the progress of the disease. In addition, armed with knowledge of the functional disturbances present, the physician is able to prescribe proper therapy and evaluate its effects. Since only one aspect of pulmonary function may be altered by some diseases, these studies may occasionally help to establish the correct diagnosis of the respiratory condition.

Although not all the tests that were described in Chapter 7 will be performed in most hospitals, and indeed, not all patients need to have the more sophisticated tests, the principles of interpretation of the tests of pulmonary function are the same. Basically, one can divide the tests into those that assess the ventilatory function of the lungs and those that are concerned with gas exchange.

VENTILATORY FUNCTION

The interpreation of tests of ventilatory function should proceed in an orderly sequential fashion. Depending on the level of sophistication of the tests that have been performed, the following sequence is recommended.

1. Is there an abnormal VC or other lung volume compartment?
2. Is there evidence of an increase in flow resistance?
3. What is the mechanism underlying these disturbances?
4. Is there evidence of maldistribution of elastic and flow resistances in the lung?

The finding of an abnormality in ventilatory function is indicative of an alteration in either the elastic or flow resistive properties of the lungs and the chest wall. However, in order to determine whether the measurements of ventilatory function (or for that matter, measurements of the elastic resistance [compliance] of the lungs and the chest wall) or the flow resistance are abnormal, they must be considered in relation to the lung volume at which they were determined. Thus we will first consider the lung volume compartments.

LUNG VOLUME

The absolute volume of the total lung capacity and its subdivisions is determined by the balance between the elastic forces and the respiratory muscles. Thus any change in lung volume compartments is indicative of either an alteration in the compliance of the lungs or chest wall, or of respiratory muscle weakness.

The vital capacity, which varies normally according to age, body size, and sex, provides a useful indication of the compliance of the respiratory apparatus, and a lower than expected VC may be indicative of a reduced distensibility. However, such an interpretation should be made with caution if the lung compartments have not been determined. Figure 8–1 illustrates that the VC may be lower than expected in patients suffering from either a restrictive disorder or an obstructive disorder. When a

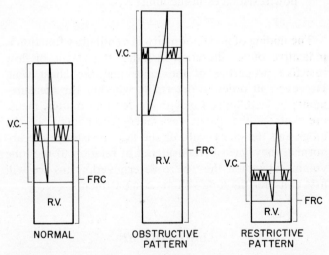

Figure 8–1. Illustrated are total lung capacity and its subdivisions when there is obstruction to air flow and when there is restriction to distention. Note that the vital capacity is lower than expected in both patterns. In the restrictive pattern the low VC is associated with a reduction in RV, FRC, and TLC. In the obstructive pattern, the low VC is associated with an increase in RV, FRC and TLC.

restrictive disorder is present the reduced VC is associated with a small TLC, whereas in the obstructive disorder the VC is low because the RV is markedly increased.

Thus if the TLC and its subdivisions are lower than expected for a given age, size, and sex, it is likely that a restrictive disorder is present. Low lung volumes may be found when the distensibility of the lungs is reduced (as in pulmonary fibrosis) or when the distensibility of the chest wall is reduced (as in kyphoscoliosis). In addition, since the determination of the subdivisions of the TLC requires voluntary effort, the TLC will be lower than expected if the respiratory muscles are weakened or paralyzed as a result of neuromuscular disease.

If the TLC or its components are greater than expected, the lungs are likely overdistended. This may be due to obstruction of the airways (as in asthma), or there may be a loss of lung recoil (as in emphysema). At one time a residual volume greater than 30 per cent of the TLC was considered to be indicative of abnormal hyperinflation. However, you will recall that the RV normally increases with age, and may be as much as 50 per cent of TLC in an elderly healthy person. In addition, it is clear that although hyperinflation is present in emphysema, the finding of hyperinflation does not mean that emphysema is present.

Finally, it is important to reiterate that a lower than expected TLC (and particularly VC) may be due to inadequate effort on the part of the patient, and may not reflect any respiratory impairment. Since several of the parameters of the TLC are derived separately, it is important to be sure that any alterations of the different subdivisions are consistent with one another before one reports that an abnormality is present.

FORCED VITAL CAPACITY

Determination of the rate at which air flows out of the lungs during the forced expiratory vital capacity maneuver (FVC) provides important information about the resistance to airflow during the forced expiration. Thus a lower than expected $FEV_{1.0}$ MMF or $\dot{V}_{max}$ 50 is suggestive of an abnormal flow resistance. An increased inspiratory resistance to airflow may also be detected by similar calculations of the forced inspiratory vital capacity curve. However, as we have seen previously, measurements of flow resistance during a forced inspiration may be less informative because a low flow rate may be related more to a lack of effort than to changes in the mechanical properties of the respiratory system.

Flow-Volume Relationship

The approach to the interpretation of the FVC can be best understood if considered in light of the relationship between the lung volume and the instantaneous flow rates during the forced expiration, i.e., the flow-volume relationship. This is illustrated in Figure 8–2, in which the flow-volume relationship (the "dynamic envelope") is plotted against the lung volume (the "static envelope") in a healthy subject. The finding of a variation from the expected flow-volume relationship, particularly the slope of the curve over the last 50 per cent of the FVC, is thought to indicate that the regional distribution of elastic and flow resistances (i.e., time constants) is unequal in the lung.

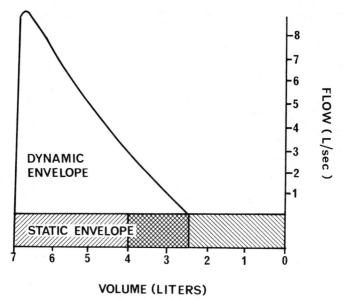

Figure 8–2. The flow–volume relationship during a forced vital capacity (FVC) maneuver is shown. The absolute lung volume is plotted on the horizontal axis (the static envelope), and the maximal expiratory flow rates during the FVC are plotted on the vertical axis (the dynamic envelope). In the example shown RV = 2.5 ℓ., FRC = 4.0 ℓ., I.C. = 3.0 ℓ., VC = 4.5 ℓ., and TLC = 7.0 ℓ.

PATTERNS OF VENTILATORY ABNORMALITY

Table 8–1 compares the patterns of abnormality of lung volume and the FVC in patients suffering from a restrictive pulmonary disorder and in those with an obstructive pulmonary disorder. The $FEV_{1.0}$, MMF, and maximum expiratory flow rates are sharply reduced in emphysema and other diseases characterized by airflow obstruction. On the other hand, these parameters may

Table 8-1   DISTURBANCES OF VENTILATORY
FUNCTION IN OBSTRUCTIVE AND
RESTRICTIVE DISEASE

TEST	OBSTRUCTIVE DISEASE	RESTRICTIVE DISEASE
VC	↔ ↓	↓ ↓
$FEV_{1.0}$	↓ ↓	↔ ↓
MMF	↓ ↓	↔ ↓
MBC	↓ ↓	↔ ↓
RV	↑ ↑	↓ ↓
FRC	↑ ↑	↓ ↓
TLC	↑ ↑	↓ ↓

also be lower than expected in patients suffering from
a restrictive disorder, such as pulmonary fibrosis, even
though there is actually no alteration in flow resistance.

Restrictive Ventilatory Pattern

As is indicated in Figure 8–3, the finding of a low
MMF or expiratory flow rates in a patient suffering from
a restrictive disorder such as pulmonary fibrosis, obesity,
or kyphoscoliosis, or in a patient whose respiratory
muscles are unable to perform normally because of a
neuromuscular disease or paralysis, can be explained by
the reduction in lung volume. It can be seen that the
expiratory flow rates, though low in absolute terms, may
actually be higher than expected at the particular lung
volume because the elastic retractive force is greater
than normal. As a corollary, it is clear that if the flow rate
is not higher than expected when the lung volume is
reduced (presumably because of a low compliance), one
can infer that the resistance to airflow is probably increased.

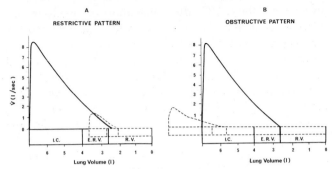

Figure 8–3. Flow–volume relationships in patients demonstrating a restrictive pattern (A) and an obstructive pattern (B) are graphed. The expected values in both patients are the same as that of the healthy subject illustrated in Figure 8–2. The observed values are indicated by the interrupted lines. In the restrictive pattern the static and dynamic envelopes are reduced, but the flow rates are consistent with the fact that the lung volume is reduced. In the obstructive pattern, the dynamic envelope is again reduced but the static envelope is increased. Here the flow rates are considerably less than expected at the increased lung volume.

Obstructive Ventilatory Pattern

The findings of a lower than normal $FEV_{1.0}$, MMF or expiratory flow rates, and an increase in TLC, FRC, and RV are indicative of airflow obstruction and overdistention of the lungs. This is illustrated in Figure 8–3, in which it can be seen that the expiratory flow rates are considerably lower than expected at equivalent lung volumes.

Post-Bronchodilator Studies

In order to determine whether the administration of a nebulized bronchodilator to a patient will result in im-

provement, the FVC after inhalation of the broncho-
dilating agent must be compared with that obtained before the bronchodilator. The effect of the bronchodilator
on the FVC in a patient suffering from diffuse bronchial
obstruction is illustrated in Figure 8–4. It is important to
point out that if the comparison is not made at equivalent
lung volumes, the MMF or flow rates at 50 per cent or
25 per cent of VC may appear to be unchanged following
the inhalation of bronchodilator. Clearly then, interpretation of the benefit, or lack of it, of a nebulized bronchodilator can be valid only if the flow rates in a particular
individual are compared at equivalent lung volumes.

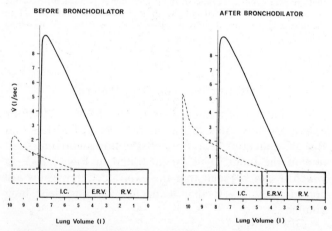

Figure 8–4. The effect of a nebulized bronchodilator on the flow-
volume relationships in a patient with obstruction to air flow. Note
that following the bronchodilator, the VC has increased (and RV decreased), the dynamic envelope has increased, and flow rates are higher
at equivalent lung volumes.

PULMONARY MECHANICS

As we have seen, the FVC and the compartments of the lung volume will usually allow for differentiation of a restrictive from an obstructive disorder. However, occasionally this is difficult, and it may be necessary to assess the mechanical properties of the lung in order to elucidate the underlying mechanism and, in some instances, the appropriate diagnosis. In addition, the assessment of pulmonary mechanics allows one to determine whether overdistention and low expiratory flow rates are due to an increased airway resistance or a loss of lung recoil. The most important determination in this regard is the assessment of the static elastic recoil of the lungs.

STATIC LUNG ELASTIC RECOIL

From the plot of the relationship between the static trans-pulmonary pressure and the lung volume (i.e., static pressure-volume curve) it is possible to determine whether a restrictive disorder is due to a lung disorder, or whether an obstructive disorder is due to airway disease or a loss of lung elastic recoil. In order to correct for differences in body size and for alterations in the pressure-volume relationship that develop as a result of disease, the volume axis is usually expressed as a per cent of the predicted TLC.

In Figure 8–5 examples of the pressure-volume relationships that are found in pulmonary disease are depicted. If the pressure-volume curve is shifted downward and to the right when compared with that of a healthy

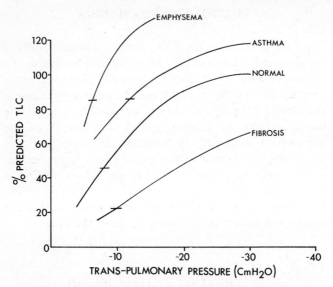

Figure 8–5. Static pressure–volume relationship of the lung in a healthy individual and in patients suffering from pulmonary fibrosis, asthma, and emphysema is shown. Note that the curve is shifted down and to the right (a given lung volume is associated with a higher pressure) in the patient with fibrosis, and up and to the left (a given lung volume is associated with a lower pressure) in asthma and emphysema. In asthma the slope of the curve is unchanged, whereas in emphysema the slope is increased.

individual, a restrictive disorder of the lungs such as fibrosis is present. If the curve is shifted upward and to the left, it may be due to an airway disease such as asthma or emphysema. However, it will be noted that the shift of the curve is less severe in asthma, the slope of the curve being essentially the same as that in a healthy individual. In emphysema, on the other hand, the slope of the curve is also altered (i.e., compliance of the lung is increased).

FLOW RESISTANCE

The finding of an increase in airway resistance by body plethysmography or an increase in total flow resistance when the mechanics of breathing are studied is indicative of an increase in resistance to airflow. On the other hand, as was pointed out earlier, it is important that these measurements be related to the lung volume at which they were determined, and an increased flow resistance should be reported only if it is different from the expected at an equivalent lung volume.

INTERACTION BETWEEN ELASTIC AND FLOW RESISTANCE

Clearly, since the level of the flow resistance is related to the lung volume, it is also related to the elastic recoil pressure of the lung. As we saw in Chapter 2, the relationship between flow resistance and lung volume is curvilinear, and the relationship of its reciprocal (flow/pressure or **airway conductance**) to lung volume is virtually linear. Thus in most clinical laboratories interpretation is based on the airway conductance per unit volume, or **specific conductance.**

Dynamic Compliance

As we have learned, the resistance to airflow in the peripheral portions of the airways (i.e., those less than 2 mm in diameter) may be markedly increased, and yet the commonly employed indices of flow resistance such as $FEV_{1.0}$, MMF, and even the airway resistance measurement itself may be within normal limits. However, when there is some obstruction in these small airways, the distribution of mechanical time constants in the lung is frequently altered, particularly when the respiratory frequency is increased, and this is reflected in measurements of the dynamic compliance of the lungs.

If the dynamic compliance of the lungs falls below 80 per cent of the static compliance at an equivalent lung volume it is considered to be frequency-dependent, and indicative of a maldistribution of the time constants within the lung (i.e., the product of the compliance and flow resistance of each unit). When frequency dependence of compliance is present but airway resistance and spirometric measurements such as the $FEV_{1.0}$ are normal, it is considered that small airway disease is present.

Upstream Resistance

Measurements of $\dot{V}_{max}$ at low lung volumes may also yield valuable information about the elastic and flow resistances. A lower than expected $\dot{V}_{max}$ may be due to an increased upstream resistance (i.e., in airways distal to the EPP) or a lower than expected driving pressure (i.e., less than expected lung elastic recoil). The relationship between the static elastic recoil pressure and $\dot{V}_{max}$ (Fig. 8–6) allows for the elucidation of the underlying cause(s) of the low flow rates. When the static pressure/flow curve is shifted to the right (i.e., pressure per unit flow is greater), the upstream resistance is increased. However, when the static pressure/flow curve falls within the expected or normal limits, the low $\dot{V}_{max}$ is due to the loss of elastic recoil. Clearly there may be situations in which a low V_{max} is due to both disturbances, which would be the interpretation if the curve is

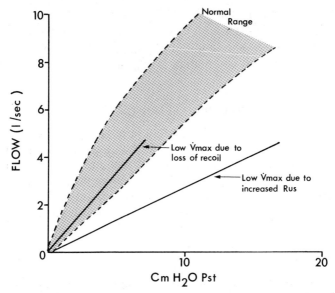

Figure 8–6. The graph shows the relationship between the static elastic recoil pressure of the lung (P_{st}) and air flow ($\dot{V}_{max}$ determined during an FVC). The stippled area represents the range in healthy individuals. Note that the $\dot{V}_{max}$ is lower than normal when there is a loss of lung elastic recoil (the pressure–flow relationships are normal, but the driving pressure is reduced), or there is an increased upstream resistance (R_{us}), i.e., a given flow rate is associated with a greater than normal pressure.

shifted to the right and the maximum static pressure is lower than expected.

Air-Helium Flow-Volume Curves

A failure of $\dot{V}_{max}$ to increase normally at almost all lung volumes when an FVC is performed after a helium-oxygen gas mixture has been breathed suggests an increase in the length of the airway segment where laminar flow is predominant (i.e., in the smaller airways). Thus when the difference in $\dot{V}_{max}$ at 50 per cent of VC ($\Delta\dot{V}_{max}$ 50) is less than expected, it is considered that "small airways" obstruction is present.

Distribution of Inspired Gas

The finding of an abnormality in tests of gas distribution such as the mixing efficiency, index of intrapulmonary mixing, or the single breath nitrogen curve is indicative of regional variations of mechanical time constants (i.e., the mechanical resistance offered by the lung, the airways, and the extrapulmonary structures).

Slope of Phase III

It has been suggested that the slope of the alveolar plateau (phase III) of the single breath nitrogen curve is primarily influenced by the elastic properties of the air spaces, but the fact that it improves following the cessation of smoking suggests that airways probably also play a role in any alterations of the slope of the plateau.

Closing Volume and Closing Capacity

The closing volume (CV) and closing capacity (CC) are nonspecific tests that are affected by both airway and parenchymal changes. An increase in the CV/VC or CC/TLC ratios suggests that there has been premature airway closure, which in turn may be due to narrowing of the lumen of small bronchioles, as in bronchitis, or a loss of radial traction on the airways, as in emphysema.

CHEMICAL REGULATION OF VENTILATION

RESPONSE TO CARBON DIOXIDE

The finding of a lower than normal ventilatory response to inhaled carbon dioxide suggests that the sensitivity of the central chemosensitive areas is diminished. However, the fact that the response of a normal subject is reduced when breathing through an artificial airway obstruction, and that it increases following the inhalation of a bronchodilator in a patient with chronic obstructive airway disease indicates that a reduced ventilatory response may be merely another reflection of ventilatory impairment, so that an impaired sensitivity need not be implicated. On the other hand, the finding of a lower than expected increase in $P_{0.1}$ (the mouth occlusion pressure developed in the first 100 milliseconds after inspiration is initiated from FRC) in response to a rising P_{CO_2} suggests that the responsiveness of the respiratory center may be diminished.

RESPONSE TO HYPOXEMIA

Like the responses to carbon dioxide, lower than expected responses to hypoxemia suggest that the chemical responsiveness is diminished, this time in the peripheral chemoreceptors. However, the possibility that a diminished response to hypoxemia is due to ventilatory impairment rather than an alteration of chemoreceptor sensitivity must once again be considered.

GAS EXCHANGE

The approach to the interpretation of tests of gas exchange and arterial blood gas tensions should be orderly and, depending on the parameters that have been measured, should follow a certain sequence that attempts to answer a series of questions:

1. Was the subject in a steady state when the blood was drawn?
2. Is the $P_{a_{O_2}}$ lower than expected for the subject's age?
3. Is the $P_{a_{CO_2}}$ abnormal?
4. Is the alveolo-arterial P_{O_2} gradient $(P(A\text{-}a)_{O_2})$ greater than expected?
5. Is the hydrogen ion concentration abnormal?
6. What is the underlying cause of any disturbance of gas exchange or acid-base balance?

STEADY STATE

In most instances arterial blood is sampled without the simultaneous collection of gas. Under these circumstances it must be inferred that the patient was resting quietly for a period before the blood was drawn and was in a steady state when it was drawn, so that abnormal blood gas tensions are a valid reflection of a disturbance in gas exchange. However, if expired gas was collected simultaneously with an arterial blood sample, the level of the respiratory quotient (R) will indicate whether the subject was in a steady state when the blood was drawn. If the R is lower than 0.65 the patient was probably hypoventilating while the blood was being drawn, and the finding of a low P_{O_2} and elevated P_{CO_2} could be the result of breath-holding or shallow respirations during the sampling. If the R is greater than 0.95, the patient was probably hyperventilating while blood was being drawn,

Table 8–2 DISTURBANCES OF GAS EXCHANGE

PARAMETER	ALVEOLAR HYPOVENTILATION		$\dot{V}/\dot{Q}$ ABNORMALITY		VENOUS ADMIXTURE	DIFFUSION DEFECT
	(a)	(b)	(c)	(d)	(e)	(f)
$\dot{V}_E$	↔↑	↓↓	↑	↑	↑↔	↑
V_D	↑↑	↔	↑	↔	↔	↔
V_D/V_T	↑↑	↑↑	↑	↔	↔	↔
$P(A\text{-}a)_{O_2}$	↔	↔	↑↑	↑↑	↑↑	↑↑
$P_{a_{O_2}}$ (room air)	↓↓	↓↓	↔↓	↓↓	↓↓	↓↓
$P_{a_{O_2}}$ (O_2)	>500	>500	>500	>500	<500	>500
$P_{a_{CO_2}}$	↑↑	↑↑	↓↔	↑↔	↓↔	↓↔

and the P_{O_2} may be slightly higher and the P_{CO_2} lower than those present under ordinary circumstances. In both circumstances, then, the status of the $P_{a_{O_2}}$ and $P_{a_{CO_2}}$ will not necessarily be indicative of the adequacy of gas exchange, and abnormal values should be interpreted with caution.

Bearing these considerations in mind, the finding of a low $P_{a_{O_2}}$ with or without an abnormal P_{CO_2} is indicative of an abnormality of gas exchange. The lower than expected $P_{a_{O_2}}$ may be due to alveolar hypoventilation, a mismatching of ventilation and perfusion within the lung, true venous admixture, a diffusion defect, or a combination of these disturbances. The salient features of these disturbances are illustrated in Table 8–2.

ALVEOLAR HYPOVENTILATION

When the $P_{a_{CO_2}}$ is elevated (hypercapnia) in association with a lower than expected $P_{a_{O_2}}$, it means that the alveolar ventilation is unable to cope with the CO_2 production, i.e., alveolar hypoventilation. This situation arises whenever the work of breathing or total body metabolism is disproportionately high for a given alveolar ventilation (as may occur in obesity), or there is excessive dead-space-like or wasted ventilation (as is found in emphysema), or the minute ventilation falls (as in barbiturate poisoning or muscular paralysis) (Table 8–2a and b).

In pure alveolar hypoventilation there is still normal equilibration of oxygen between the alveoli and the pulmonary capillary blood so that the $P(A-a)_{O_2}$ is not abnormal. Thus the findings of a low $P_{a_{O_2}}$, a high $P_{a_{CO_2}}$ and a normal $P(A-a)_{O_2}$ are indicative of uncomplicated alveolar hypoventilation. However, if the A-a gradient is found to be increased when the P_{CO_2} is elevated, additional physiologic disturbances must be present.

ALVEOLO-ARTERIAL P_{O_2} GRADIENT

In healthy young individuals the alveolar to arterial (A-a) P_{O_2} gradient is usually less than 10 torr when breathing room air, and it increases with age as the arterial P_{O_2} falls. The finding of a $P(A-a)_{O_2}$ that is greater than expected for a given age is indicative of the presence of one or more of the other three physiologic disturbances.

MISMATCHING OF VENTILATION AND PERFUSION

Mismatching of the regional ventilation and perfusion in the lungs accounts for the major proportion of the $P(A-a)_{O_2}$ in both healthy and diseased lungs. Blood leaving well ventilated alveoli may be poorly perfused (i.e., the ventilation/perfusion ratio is high), or poorly ventilated alveoli may continue to be well perfused (i.e., the ventilation/perfusion ratio is low).

Dead-Space-Like Ventilation

The dead space/tidal volume ratio (V_D/V_T) is normally less than 30 per cent in young individuals, and rises to about 40 per cent in older subjects. A ratio that is greater than expected indicates that there are ventilated alveoli that have limited perfusion or, in the extreme case, are not perfused. The gas entering these alveoli takes little part, if any, in gas exchange, and the gas concentrations are virtually the same as those inspired ("dead-space-like ventilation"). The blood leaving these alveoli is fully oxygenated and often excessively depleted of carbon dioxide, so that the $P_{a_{O_2}}$ may be relatively normal and the $P_{a_{CO_2}}$ may be normal or low (Table 8–2c). However, the $P(A-a)_{O_2}$ will be elevated under these circumstances.

Venous-Admixture-Like Perfusion

Blood leaving inadequately ventilated alveoli or, in the extreme case, nonventilated alveoli (i.e., a low ventilation/perfusion ratio) will be only slightly aerated, if at all. This poorly aerated blood will mix with the "arterialized blood" coming from well ventilated, well perfused alveoli, so that the $P_{a_{O_2}}$ will be low and the $P_{a_{CO_2}}$ slightly elevated (Table 8–2d). In most cases there is sufficient hyperventilation of other well perfused alveoli, so the $P_{a_{CO_2}}$ is usually normal or even low. However, the hyperventilation does not lead to significant correction of the hypoxemia because of the shape of the oxyhemoglobin dissociation curve.

TRUE VENOUS ADMIXTURE

Even in healthy individuals a small part of the $P(A-a)_{O_2}$ is due to the admixture of venous blood into the systemic arterial blood via the thebesian and the bronchial veins, which empty into the left side of the heart, and the pulmonary veins. There is an increase in true venous admixture in certain congenital heart diseases, and when there are abnormal pulmonary arteriovenous communications. The $P_{a_{CO_2}}$ is usually below the normal limits in this situation because the hypoxemia frequently stimulates an increase in ventilation.

Failure of the $P_{a_{O_2}}$ to rise above 500 torr while 100 per cent oxygen is being breathed suggests the presence of a greater than normal amount of true venous admixture (Table 8–2e). However, it is important to recognize that the $P_{a_{O_2}}$ may not rise sufficiently when there is significant polycythemia, even when there is no increase in true venous admixture. In addition, continued perfusion of lung regions that are not ventilated at all, because of obstruction, collapse, pulmonary edema, or consolidation, will produce a picture much like true venous admixture. Under these circumstances the intravenous injection of a marker such as green dye (as is used to determine cardiac output) may help to delineate the disturbance. The dye will appear in a peripheral artery within a normal period of time if the venous admixture is due to the perfusion of non-ventilated areas, and will appear earlier than expected if it is due to true venous admixture.

DIFFUSION ABNORMALITY

The finding of a low diffusing capacity is usually a reflection of the mismatching of ventilation and perfusion throughout the lungs, rather than a diffusion defect. Thus a low $D_{L_{CO}}$ is usually merely a reflection of abnormal gas exchange. Nevertheless, a diffusion defect may develop in some patients during heavy exercise and play a major role in increasing the $P(A\text{-}a)_{O_2}$. A true diffusion anormality may occur when the area of alveolar surface available for diffusion is reduced. This can occur as a result of structural changes in the terminal lung units (as in diffuse pulmonary fibrosis or the late stages of emphysema), or following the operative removal of considerable lung tissue. When a diffusion abnormality is present the low $P_{a_{O_2}}$ is often associated with a low $P_{a_{CO_2}}$ (Table 8–2f).

The $D_{L_{CO}}$ may be falsely low if the alveolar carbon monoxide concentration has been inaccurately estimated. However, if the carbon monoxide extraction is also low, the low $D_{L_{CO}}$ indicates either a mismatching of ventilation and perfusion or a reduction of the effective internal surface area of the lung available for gas transfer.

TISSUE HYPOXIA

Before leaving the subject of gas exchange it is important to point out that the interpretation should concern itself not just with the level of the arterial blood gas tensions, but with the adequacy of tissue oxygenation. We have dealt mainly with hypoxemia (a lower than normal oxygen tension or saturation in the arterial blood) till now. Although hypoxemia is one cause of tissue hypoxia, other factors involved in oxygen transport are equally important. Since oxygen is transported mainly in combination with hemoglobin, the level of the hemoglobin and the amount of blood coming to the tissues (i.e., cardiac output) are important determinants of the adequacy of the oxygen supply to the tissues. Thus when severe anemia is present, the hemoglobin is altered as in carbon monoxide poisoning, or in the critically ill patient in shock, and severe hypoxia may be present even though the $P_{a_{O_2}}$ is maintained within normal limits. Although cardiac output may be measured directly, many clinicians now utilize the mixed venous oxygen content ($C_{\bar{v}_{O_2}}$) as an indicator of the adequacy of the cardiac output ($\dot{Q}$) and overall tissue oxygenation. This is deduced from the Fick Equation.

$$\dot{Q} = \frac{\dot{V}_{O_2}}{C_{a_{O_2}} - C_{\bar{v}_{O_2}}}$$

$$\dot{Q}\,(C_{a_{O_2}} - C_{\bar{v}_{O_2}}) = \dot{V}_{O_2}$$

The $C_{a_{O_2}}$ can be derived from the $P_{a_{O_2}}$ and the Hb, and $\dot{V}_{O_2}$ is considered relatively constant. Under such circumstances and because $C_{a_{O_2}}$ is usually maintained at a constant level, the changes in the $C_{\bar{v}_{O_2}}$ are a good reflection of the level of the cardiac output and overall tissue oxygenation. Clearly one cannot draw any conclusions about a particular organ or tissue because the various tissues extract different amounts of oxygen.

ACID-BASE BALANCE

The characteristic picture found in the blood in the acid-base disorders that are encountered clinically is illustrated in Figure 8–7, whereas the underlying mechanisms and clinical examples are presented in Table 8–3 (respiratory disturbances) and Table 8–4 (metabolic disturbances).

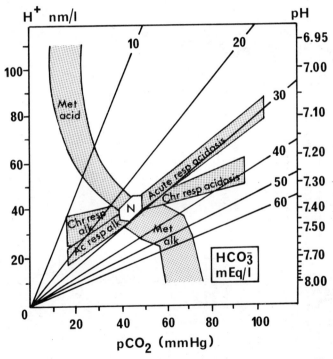

Figure 8–7. This figure shows the relationship between $P_{a_{CO_2}}$, pH, and H^+ concentration, and the alterations seen in respiratory and metabolic disorders of acid-base balance.

Table 8–3 RESPIRATORY DISORDERS OF ACID-BASE BALANCE

DISORDER	GENERAL MECHANISM	SPECIFIC MECHANISM	EXAMPLES	BLOOD PICTURE
Respiratory acidosis	Inadequate alveolar ventilation relative to carbon dioxide production	Airway obstruction	Upper airway, large airways, COPD, asthma	$P_{a_{CO_2}}$ high
		Respiratory center depression	Brain disease, primary?; administration of anesthetics, narcotics, sedatives; chronic CO_2 retention; compensation for metabolic alkalosis	pH low — HCO_3^- normal (acute) high (compensated)
		Neuromuscular impairment	Myopathies, neuropathies, administration of muscle relaxants	Cl low if compensated K normal or high
		Chest wall disease	Kyphoscoliosis, obesity, tight binders, etc.	
Respiratory alkalosis	Increased alveolar ventilation relative to carbon dioxide production	Exogenous administration of respiratory stimulants Iatrogenic	Salicylates, progesterone Excessive mechanical ventilation	$P_{a_{CO_2}}$ low pH high
		Increased respiratory center activity	Psychogenic (emotion), brain disease, fever, arterial hypoxemia, reflex from lung receptors?; compensation for metabolic acidosis	HCO_3^- normal (acute) low if compensated Cl high K low

ASSESSMENT OF ACID-BASE STATUS

The analysis of the acid-base status in the body from an arterial blood sample can be approached in many ways. Whichever approach is adopted, it should proceed in an orderly fashion. A relatively simple approach is to start with the pH.

If an acidemia is present (pH < 7.35) one must then determine whether the primary disturbance is respiratory or metabolic. If the $P_{a_{CO_2}}$ is greater than 45 torr, a respiratory acidosis is present, and if it is between 35 and 45 torr, a metabolic acidosis is present.

If an alkalemia is present (pH > 7.45) one must again determine whether the primary disturbance is respiratory or metabolic. If the $P_{a_{CO_2}}$ is less than 35 torr, a respiratory alkalosis is present, and if it is between 35 and 45 torr, a metabolic alkalosis is present.

If the pH is normal (between 7.35 and 7.45) but the $P_{a_{CO_2}}$ and HCO_3^- are abnormal, the acid-base disturbance is chronic and somewhat more difficult to define. On the whole, compensatory processes do not return the pH to normal, but if it is within the normal range and the $P_{a_{CO_2}}$ and HCO_3^- are abnormal, the alteration in acid-base balance is the result of several disturbances. In such cases, proper clinical evaluation and elucidation of the duration of the alteration, and the therapy the patient has been receiving may be the only guides to the major defect present. However, the level of the pH will once again provide a valuable clue about the disturbance that is present. Thus if the pH is near the lower limits of "normality," the major disturbance present is probably an acidosis, whereas if it is near the upper limit of the normal range, the major disturbance is probably an alkalosis.

Table 8-4 METABOLIC DISORDERS OF ACID-BASE BALANCE

DISORDER	GENERAL MECHANISM	SPECIFIC MECHANISM	EXAMPLES	BLOOD PICTURE
	Gain of strong acid by extracellular fluid	Exogenous agents that induce hyperchloremic acidosis	NH$_4$Cl, argenine chloride, lysine, HCl, acetazolamide	
		Exogenous agents that lead to production of endogenous acids	Salicylates, ethylene glycol, methyl alcohol	HCO$_3^-$ low
		Increased production of non-volatile acids due to incomplete oxidation of fat	Diabetic ketoacidosis, starvation, alcoholism (acute and chronic)	pH low
Metabolic acidosis		Increased production of non-volatile acids due to incomplete oxidation of carbohydrate (anaerobic metabolism) —lactate acidosis	Primary lactate acidosis (idiopathic, or in association with leukemia, diabetes, and liver disease; circulatory insufficiency (drug induced — phenformin)	P$_{a_{CO_2}}$ normal (acute) low as compensation
	Loss of HCO$_3^-$ from the extracellular fluid	Via kidreys	Acute and chronic renal failure, renal tubular acidosis, compensation for respiratory alkalosis	Cl normal or high K high, unless associated with K depletion
		Via intestines	Diarrhea or loss of small intestinal alkaline content	

Metabolic alkalosis	Gain of HCO_3^- from the extracellular fluid	Excess alkali intake	Ingestion of absorbable antacids ($NaHCO_3$), infusion of alkali; milk-alkali syndrome	HCO_3^- high pH high
		Oxidation of salts of weak organic acids	Ingestion or infusion of lactate, citrate, or acetate	
		Via kidneys	Compensation for respiratory acidosis	
	Loss of acid from the extracellular fluid	Loss of HCl	Vomiting, gastric suction, diarrhea, gastrocolic fistula	$P_{a_{CO_2}}$ normal (acute) slightly elevated as compensation
		Potassium depletion	Diuretics, vomiting, diarrhea, fistulas, low intake, steroid therapy, Cushing's syndrome, primary aldosteronism, potassium-losing enteropathy, potassium-losing nephropathy	Cl low K usually low

In some laboratories the acid-base state of the patient is reported in terms of "base excess" or "base deficit." However, these terms simply indicate that base has been added to or lost from the extracellular fluid, and they are of no help in determining the mechanism responsible for the gain or loss of base. Clearly a "base excess" will be present in both a metabolic alkalosis and a compensated respiratory acidosis. In addition, since the base excess or deficit is estimated from an in vitro test, the values obtained are different from those that would be obtained if it were possible to carry out the test in vivo.

In some cases, calculation of the unmeasured anions (the anion gap) is helpful in establishing the cause of a metabolic acidosis. This is determined by subtracting the sum of the plasma bicarbonate and chloride levels from the plasma sodium concentration. If the anion gap is less than 12 mM/liter (hyperchloremic acidosis), the acidosis is probably due to the intestinal loss of bicarbonate or the administration of ammonium chloride, arginine chloride lysine, or acetazolomide. An anion gap greater than 12 mM/liter is typical of an increased production of non-volatile acids (as in renal failure) and poisoning by salicylates, ethylene glycol, and methyl alcohol.

EXERCISE RESPONSE

The assessment of certain parameters of function during exercise provides information regarding exercise capacity and the factors that may limit it. In order to identify the possible mechanisms involved in limiting exercise performance, it is essential to recognize that many cardiopulmonary parameters are altered during exercise, even in healthy individuals. Thus oxygen consumption ($\dot{V}_{O_2}$), carbon dioxide production ($\dot{V}_{CO_2}$), respiratory quotient (R), ventilation ($\dot{V}_E$)—both V_T and f, physiologic dead space (V_D), cardiac output, blood lactate level, and the arteriovenous O_2 content difference all increase. On the other hand, the V_D/V_T ratio (i.e., dead-space-like ventilation) and venous-admixture-like perfusion decrease, while the $P(A-a)_{O_2}$ and arterial blood gas tensions are little altered when healthy individuals undertake moderately heavy exercise.

A variety of mechanisms, both respiratory and non-respiratory, may limit exercise performance in patients. Table 8–5 indicates that there are certain alterations of gas exchange parameters during exercise when the individual is physically unfit, while other disturbances are encountered when there is cardiovascular or respiratory impairment. Only if none of these abnormal responses to exercise occur should one entertain the' diagnosis of psychogenic dyspnea.

Table 8–5   GAS EXCHANGE ABNORMALITIES DURING EXERCISE

PARAMETER	CARDIO-VASCULAR IMPAIRMENT OR PHYSICAL UNFITNESS	VENTILATORY IMPAIRMENT	$\dot{V}/\dot{Q}$ IMBALANCE	
	(a)	(b)	(c)	(d)
$\dot{V}_E$ rise	↑	↑	↑	↑
R	↑↑	↓↔	↔	↔
V_D/V_T (%)	←↑↓	↓↔	↓	↑
$P(A-a)_{O_2}$	↓↔	↔	↑↑	↑↑
$P_{a_{O_2}}$	↔↓	↓↓	↓↓	↓↓
$P_{a_{CO_2}}$	↔↓	↑↑	↔↓	↔↑
pH	↓↓	↓↓	↔↑	↔↑

If, during moderate exercise, the respiratory quotient rises and acidemia develops (due to the accumulation of lactate), it means that the oxygen delivery is unable to meet the energy demands of the exercising muscles. Table 8–5a indicates that this will occur if the cardio-vascular system is unable to cope with the increased demands of the tissues during the exercise, or if the individual is not physically fit.

A fall in $P_{a_{O_2}}$ and a rise in $P_{a_{CO_2}}$ during the exercise indicates that the patient is unable to increase alveolar ventilation sufficiently during the exercise load to cope with the increased metabolic production of carbon dioxide (Table 8–5b). Thus these findings suggest that exercise performance is limited by ventilatory impairment.

If the $P_{a_{O_2}}$ rises and the $P(A\text{-}a)_{O_2}$ falls during exercise (Table 8–5c), this indicates that the diffusion of oxygen is not impaired and that the matching of ventilation and perfusion throughout the lungs has improved during exercise as a result of the increased ventilation of areas of lung with a low ventilation/perfusion ratio.

Conversely, if the $P_{a_{O_2}}$ falls and the $P(A\text{-}a)_{O_2}$ widens during the exercise (Table 8–5d), it can be inferred that the exercise resulted in a greater defect in oxygen transfer due to either increased mismatching of the blood and gas distribution in the lungs, or a diffusion defect.

SELF-ASSESSMENT
Patient Examples

1. A 60 year old woman (a non-smoker) was admitted to hospital with an 8 week history of progressive increase of a cough that produced 1/4 cup of mucopurulent sputum/day, feverishness, increasing dyspnea, and fatigue as well as a loss of 7 pounds in weight. There was no history of allergies, chest pain, wheezing, or swelling of the ankles or joints.

On physical examination, the respiratory frequency was 24/min. Chest movement and air entry were diminished bilaterally, and there were mid and late inspiratory crepitations over the entire chest.

The pressure-volume characteristics were determined and are shown in Figure 8–8, while ventilatory function studies provided the following data:

Parameter	VC	RV	FRC	TLC	MMF	$\dot{V}_{peak}$	$\dot{V}_{max}50$	$\dot{V}_{max}25$
Predicted	2.79	1.41	2.19	4.20	2.85	5.53	2.76	1.60
Observed	1.51	0.75	1.34	2.26	1.13	2.06	1.10	0.49

From these studies one can say that
a. elastic recoil is _____
   (1) normal.   (2) diminished.   (3) increased.

b. airway conductance is probably _____
   (1) normal.   (2) diminished.   (3) increased.

c. the studies are indicative of _____
   (1) normality.
   (2) a restrictive pattern.
   (3) an obstructive pattern.
   (4) a mixed pattern.

d. The arterial blood findings that would best fit the ventilatory function findings are

	$P_{a_{O_2}}$	$P_{a_{CO_2}}$	pH
(1)	85	40	7.12
(2)	45	23	7.52
(3)	45	65	7.29

After therapy was instituted the ventilatory function studies were repeated.

Parameter	VC	RV	FRC	TLC	MMF	$\dot{V}_{peak}$	$\dot{V}_{max}50$	$\dot{V}_{max}25$
Predicted	2.79	1.41	2.19	4.2	2.85	5.53	2.76	1.60
Observed	2.75	1.35	1.90	4.1	2.30	5.35	2.10	0.95

e. The elastic recoil is probably _____
   (1) normal.   (2) diminished.   (3) increased.

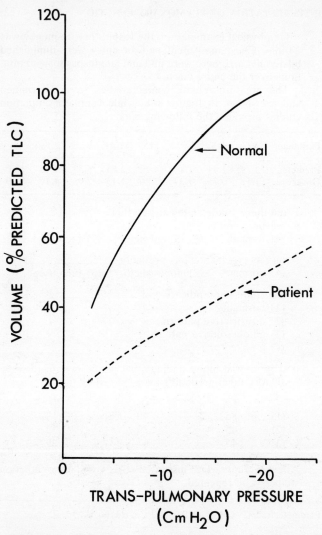

Figure 8–8. The pressure volume characteristics in a 60 year old female patient and those of a healthy female of similar age are shown on the graph.

226

f. The airway conductance is probably _____
   (1) normal.   (2) diminished.   (3) increased.

g. The data now indicate _____
   (1) normality.
   (2) a restrictive pattern.
   (3) an obstructive pattern.
   (4) a mixed pattern.

2. In 3 patients the following measurements were made when the barometric pressure was 747 torr.

Parameter		A	B	C
$\dot{V}_E$ (ℓ/min)		12.	9.	12.
f (no/min)		25	20	25
$P_{a_{O_2}}$	while breathing air	52	52	52
$P_{a_{CO_2}}$		36	72	32
$F_{E_{CO_2}}$		0.04	0.04	0.03
$P_{a_{O_2}}$	while breathing 100%	550	510	400
$P_{a_{CO_2}}$	O_2	34	80	35
$D_{L_{CO}}$ (% pred.)		98	98	98

For each patient
a. calculate
   A-a Gradient (on air)   _____ _____ _____

   Dead space/tidal vol. ratio   _____ _____ _____

b. indicate whether the following is likely to be present (+) or absent (−)

   Respiratory alkalosis   _____ _____ _____

   Diffusion defect   _____ _____ _____

   Ventilation of poorly perfused
     alveoli   _____ _____ _____

   Alveolar hypoventilation   _____ _____ _____

Perfusion of poorly ventilated
alveoli   _____ _____ _____

True venous admixture   _____ _____ _____

Respiratory acidosis   _____ _____ _____

3. The following results were reported in a patient who was
   brought into hospital complaining of severe shortness of
   breath:

Parameter	VC	MMF	$\dot{V}_{max}50$	$\dot{V}_{max}25$	RV	FRC	TLC	$D_{L_{CO}}$
Predicted	4.00	5.0	5.2	2.50	2.0	3.45	6.00	20
Observed	1.50	2.0	1.8	1.25	1.0	1.72	2.50	18

	On Air	On O_2
$P_{a_{O_2}}$	40	520
$P_{a_{CO_2}}$	30	40
pH	7.50	7.40

a. The patient was probably suffering from _____
   (1) obstructive disease.
   (2) restrictive disease.
   (3) a combination of both.
   (4) none of the above.

b. The hypoxemia seen while the patient was breathing
   room air is probably due to _____
   (1) alveolar hypoventilation.
   (2) true right-to-left shunt.
   (3) anemia.
   (4) ventilation/perfusion imbalance.
   (5) a diffusion defect.

O_2 therapy was immediately administered with a venturi
mask (24%), and a blood sample was taken. The inspired O_2
concentration was then increased to 28% and further blood
samples were taken. The following reports were obtained:

Parameter	After 1 Hour	After 2 Hours	After 3 Hours
$P_{a_{O_2}}$	60	70	80
$P_{a_{CO_2}}$	38	40	24
pH	7.42	7.41	7.55
$F_{I_{O_2}}$	.24	.28	.28

c. These values are indicative of _____
   (1) gradual improvement in gas exchange.
   (2) deterioration in gas exchange.
   (3) no change.

d. The acid-base status after 3 hours was indicative of____
   (1) respiratory acidosis.
   (2) respiratory alkalosis.
   (3) metabolic acidosis.
   (4) metabolic alkalosis.

4. In a 9 year old girl with cystic fibrosis, arterial blood
   analysis revealed a pH of 7.25, a $P_{a_{CO_2}}$ of 75 torr, and a
   $P_{a_{O_2}}$ of 35 torr while breathing room air.

   a. The data indicates _____
      (1) respiratory acidosis with acidemia.
      (2) respiratory acidosis without acidemia.
      (3) metabolic acidosis with acidemia.
      (4) respiratory alkalosis with acidemia.
      (5) none of the above.

   b. The $P(A-a)_{O_2}$ was probably _____
      (1) normal.
      (2) less than normal.
      (3) greater than normal.

   c. The hypoxemia was probably due to _____
      (1) alveolar hypoventilation.
      (2) ventilation/perfusion imbalance.
      (3) both of the above.
      (4) anemia.
      (5) none of the above.

During 100 per cent oxygen breathing, the arterial blood analysis showed a $P_{a_{O_2}}$ of 520 torr and a $P_{a_{CO_2}}$ of 90 torr.

d. This indicates that the cause of the hypoxemia during room air breathing was not due to _____
   (1) diffusion defect.
   (2) true venous admixture.
   (3) alveolar hyperventilation.
   (4) all of the above.

After treatment for 36 hours, repeated arterial blood analysis revealed a pH of 7.58, a $P_{a_{CO_2}}$ of 44 torr, and a $P_{a_{O_2}}$ of 54 torr while the subject was breathing room air.

e. These results now indicate _____
   (1) alveolar hypoventilation.
   (2) metabolic alkalosis with alkalemia.
   (3) respiratory alkalosis with alkalemia.
   (4) respiratory acidosis.
   (5) none of the above.

f. The $P(A-a)_{O_2}$ was _____
   (1) improved.   (2) worse.   (3) unchanged.

g. The findings suggest _____
   (1) alveolar ventilation was now adequate.
   (2) ventilation/perfusion imbalance had improved.
   (3) alveolar ventilation was inadequate.
   (4) ventilation/perfusion imbalance had deteriorated.

5. In a patient admitted to hospital, the following data were obtained:

Parameter	TLC	FRC	RV	VC	$FEV_{1.0}$	MMF	$\dot{V}_{peak}$	$\dot{V}_{max}50$	$\dot{V}_{max}25$
Predicted	6.0	3.0	2.0	4.0	3.0	6.0	9.0	6.0	2.0
Observed	7.0	5.0	4.2	2.8	2.0	3.0	5.0	3.0	1.0

a. The data indicates _____
   (1) hyperinflation.
   (2) hyperventilation.
   (3) hyperpnea.
   (4) none of the above.

   b. The pattern is _____
     (1) restrictive.
     (2) obstructive.
     (3) mixed.
     (4) no disorder of function.

   c. Resistance to air flow is probably _____
     (1) increased.   (2) decreased.   (3) normal.

   d. The underlying condition could be _____
     (1) emphysema.
     (2) bronchitis.
     (3) asthma.
     (4) all of the above.
     (5) none of the above.

After a nebulized bronchodilator the following measurements were obtained:

Parameter	TLC	FRC	RV	VC	$FEV_{1.0}$	MMF	$\dot{V}_{peak}$	$\dot{V}_{max}50$	$\dot{V}_{max}25$
Observed	7.0	4.0	3.0	4.0	2.5	3.0	6.0	3.0	1.0

   e. The data indicate _____ in lung volume
     (1) improvement
     (2) deterioration
     (3) no change

   f. and _____ in airflow resistance.
     (1) improvement
     (2) deterioration
     (3) no change

   g. You would recommend that bronchodilators are _____
     (1) indicated.
     (2) not indicated.
     (3) contraindicated.

6. A patient was admitted to hospital and diagnosed as having chronic bronchitis with a superimposed respiratory infection and congestive heart failure. He was given antibiotics and diuretics. Arterial blood analysis with a

barometric pressure of 747 torr revealed $F_{I_{O_2}}$ 0.21, $P_{a_{O_2}}$ 35, $P_{a_{CO_2}}$ 55, and pH 7.26.

a. This indicated _____
   (1) metabolic alkalemia
   (2) respiratory acidemia
   (3) respiratory acidosis
   (4) metabolic alkalosis
   (5) all of the above
   (6) none of the above

b. and _____
   (1) alveolar hypoventilation.
   (2) ventilation/perfusion imbalance.
   (3) neither of these.
   (4) both of these.

The next day he developed a cardiac arrest, was resuscitated and placed on a ventilator, and the previous treatment was continued. Arterial blood analysis revealed: $F_{I_{O_2}}$ 0.21, $P_{a_{O_2}}$ 40, $P_{a_{CO_2}}$ 45, and pH 7.10.

c. This assessment now indicated _____
   (1) metabolic alkalemia
   (2) respiratory acidemia
   (3) respiratory acidosis
   (4) metabolic alkalosis
   (5) all of the above
   (6) none of the above

d. and _____
   (1) alveolar hypoventilation,
   (2) ventilation/perfusion imbalance,
   (3) neither of these,
   (4) both of these,

e. while gas exchange was _____
   (1) improved.
   (2) worse.
   (3) unchanged.

On day 3, arterial blood analysis revealed: $F_{I_{O_2}}$ 0.24, $P_{a_{O_2}}$ 50, $P_{a_{CO_2}}$ 45, and pH 7.20.

 f. This assessment now indicated _____
  (1) metabolic alkalemia
  (2) respiratory acidemia
  (3) respiratory acidosis
  (4) metabolic alkalosis
  (5) all of the above
  (6) none of the above

 g. and _____
  (1) alveolar hypoventilation,
  (2) ventilation/perfusion imbalance,
  (3) neither of these,
  (4) both of these,

 h. while gas exchange was _____
  (1) improved.
  (2) worse.
  (3) unchanged.

On day 6, arterial blood analysis revealed: $F_{I_{O_2}}$ 0.24, $P_{a_{O_2}}$ 60, $P_{a_{CO_2}}$ 40, and pH 7.46.

 i. This assessment now indicated _____
  (1) metabolic alkalemia
  (2) respiratory acidemia
  (3) respiratory acidosis
  (4) metabolic alkalosis
  (5) all of the above
  (6) none of the above

 j. and _____
  (1) alveolar hypoventilation,
  (2) ventilation/perfusion imbalance,
  (3) neither of these,
  (4) both of these,

 k. while gas exchange was _____
  (1) improved. (2) worse. (3) unchanged.

7. A 60 year old patient complaining of shortness of breath was admitted to the hospital (barometric pressure 747 torr). The following information was acquired while determining pulmonary mechanics:

	Pleural Mouth Differential Pressure (cm H_2O)	Volume Change (ml)	Flow Rate (ℓ/sec)
End-expiration	−4		
End-inspiration	−14	600	
Mid-inspiration	−11	300	2.0

Parameter	Predicted (liters)	Observed (% Pred.)
TLC	8.0	75
VC	5.0	75
ERV	1.0	100
RV	2.0	75

ARTERIAL BLOOD ANALYSIS

	On Air	On 100% O_2
$\dot{V}_E$	15.0	
f	25	
$F_{E_{N_2}}$	.80	
$F_{E_{O_2}}$	.16	
$P_{a_{O_2}}$	68	300
$P_{a_{CO_2}}$	42	40
pH	7.22	7.20
$C_{\bar{v}_{O_2}}$	5.72	9.3
$P_{c_{O_2}}$	96	
Hemoglobin	10 gm	

Circle the correct answer.

a. Lung compliance (ℓ/cm H_2O) was _____

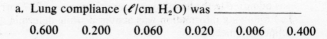

  0.600   0.200   0.060   0.020   0.006   0.400

b. Flow resistance (cm H_2O/ℓ/sec) was

    1.0   2.0   4.0   0.1   0.5   5.0

c. The disorder is probably

    restrictive   obstructive   mixed

d. RV/TLC ratio is

    1/4   1/3   1/2   1/6   1/5

e. $\dot{V}_{max}$ would be expected to be

    low   normal   high

f. $P(A\text{-}a)_{O_2}$ (torr) was

    10   15   20   25   30   35

g. V_D/V_T ratio was

    1/4   1/2   1/3   1/8   1/6   1/5

h. $\dot{V}_A$ (ℓ/min) was

    10   8   12   6   4   9

i. The hypoxemia was due to

    diffusion defect   anemia   alveolar hyperventilation

    venous admixture   alveolar hypoventilation

i. Serum bicarbonate was

    high   low   normal

k. Inspiratory capacity (ℓ) was

    1   2   3   4   5   6

l. Acid-base status indicated

    respiratory acidemia   metabolic acidemia

    respiratory acidosis   metabolic acidosis

    none of these

SUGGESTED READING

Bates, D. V., Macklem, P. T., and Christie, R. V.: Respiratory Function in Disease. Ed. 2, Philadelphia, W. B. Saunders Co., 1971.

Buist, A. S.: The single-breath nitrogen test. New Eng. J. Med., *293*: 438, 1975.

Buist, A. S., and Ross, B. B.: Predicted values for closing volumes using a modified single breath nitrogen test. Am. Rev. Respir. Dis., *107*:744, 1973.

Buist, A. S., and Ross, B. B.: Quantitative analysis of the alveolar plateau in the diagnosis of early airway obstruction. Am. Rev. Respir. Dis., *108*:1078, 1973.

Burrows, B., Knudson, R. J., and Kettel, L. J.: Respiratory Insufficiency. Chicago, Year Book Medical Publishers, 1975.

Cherniack, R. M.: Ventilatory function in normal children. C.M.A.J., *87*:80, 1962.

Cherniack, R. M., Cherniack, L., and Naimark, A.: Respiration in Health and Disease. Ed. 2, Philadelphia, W. B. Saunders Co., 1972.

Cherniack, R. M., and Raber, M.: Normal standards for ventilatory function using an automated wedge spirometer. Am. Rev. Respir. Dis., *106*:38, 1972.

Comroe, J. H., Jr.: Physiology of Respiration. Ed. 2, Chicago, Year Book Medical Publishers, 1974.

Comroe, J. H., Jr., Forster, R. E., Dubois, A. B., Briscoe, W. A., and Carlsen, E.: The Lung: Clinical Physiology and Pulmonary Function Tests. Ed. 2, Chicago, Year Book Medical Publishers, 1962.

Cotes, J. E.: Lung Function: Assessment and Application in Medicine. Ed. 2, Oxford, Blackwell Scientific Publishers, 1968.

Filley, G. F.: Acid-Base and Blood Gas Regulation. Philadelphia, Lea and Febiger, 1971.

Goldman, H. I., and Becklake, M. R.: Respiratory function tests. Normal values at medium altitudes and the prediction of normal results. Amer. Rev. Tuberc., *79*:457, 1959.

Hills, A. G.: Acid-Base Balance: Chemistry, Physiology and Pathophysiology. Baltimore, Williams and Wilkins Co., 1973.

Johnson, R. L., Jr., Spicer, W. S., Bishop, J. M., and Forster, R. E.: Pulmonary capillary blood volume, flow and diffusing capacity during exercise. J. Appl. Physiol., *15*:893, 1960.

Johnson, R. L., Jr., Taylor, H. F., and DeGraff, A. C., Jr.: Functional significance of a low pulmonary diffusing capacity for carbon monoxide. J. Clin. Invest., *44*:789, 1965.

Jones, N. L.: Exercise testing in pulmonary evaluation: rationale, methods and the normal respiratory response to exercise. New Eng. J. Med., *293*:541, 1975.

Jones, N. L.: Exercise testing in pulmonary evaluation: clinical applications. New Eng. J. Med., *293*:647, 1975.

Macklem, P. T.: Tests of lung mechanics. New Eng. J. Med., *293*:339, 1975.

Macklem, P. T., and Meade, J.: The physiological basis of common pulmonary function tests. Arch. Environ. Hlth., *14*:5, 1967.

McCarthy, D. S., Spencer, R., Green, R., and Milic-Emili, J.: Measurements of closing volume as a simple and sensitive test for early detection of small airway disease. Amer. J. Med., *52*:747, 1972.

McGrath, M. W., and Thomson, M. L.: The effect of age, body size and lung volume change on alveolar-capillary permeability and diffusing capacity in man. J. Physiol., *146*:472, 1959.

Milic-Emili, J.: Clinical methods for assessing the ventilatory response to carbon dioxide and hypoxia. New Eng. J. Med., *293*:864, 1975.

Raine, J. M., and Bishop, J. M.: A- a difference in O_2 tension and physiologic dead space in normal man. J. Appl. Physiol., *18*:284, 1963.

Refsum, H. E.: Acid-base disturbances in chronic pulmonary disease. Ann. N.Y. Acad. Sci., *133*:142, 1966.

Turner, J. M., Mead, J., and Wohl, M. E.: Elasticity of human lungs in relation to age. J. Appl. Physiol., *25*:664, 1968.

West, J. B.: Respiratory Physiology: The Essentials. Baltimore, Williams and Wilkins Co., 1974.

Woolcock, A. J., Vincent, N. J., and Macklem, P. T.: Frequency dependence of compliance as a test for obstruction in small airways. J. Clin. Invest., *48*:1097, 1969.

Appendix I

NORMAL STANDARDS

Table 1 PREDICTION EQUATIONS FOR SPIROMETRY IN CHILDREN

PARAMETER	MALE	FEMALE
FVC*	$0.05134 \times A + .04053 \times H - 3.655$	$0.09096 \times A + .02786 \times H - 2.554$
$FEV_{1.0}$†	$0.0335 \times H - 2.855$	$0.0291 \times H - 2.482$
MMF*	$0.0259 \times A + 0.02792 \times H - 1.75$	$0.0647 \times A + 0.01982 \times H - 1.08$

*Cherniack, R. M.: Ventilatory function in normal children. C.M.A.J., 89:80, 1962.
†Dickman, M. L., et al.: Spirometric standard for normal children and adolescents (ages 5 years through 18 years). Am. Rev. Respir. Dis., 104:680, 1971.
A = age in years
H = height in centimeters

Table 2. PREDICTION EQUATIONS FOR LUNG VOLUME IN CHILDREN

PARAMETER	MALE	FEMALE
TLC	$5.6 \times 10^{-6} \times (H)^{2.67}$	$4.0 \times 10^{-6} \times (H)^{2.73}$
FRC	$7.50 \times 10^{-7} \times (H)^{2.92}$	$1.78 \times 10^{-6} \times (H)^{2.74}$
RV	$4.41 \times 10^{-6} \times (H)^{2.41}$	$4.41 \times 10^{-6} \times (H)^{2.41}$

Polgar, G., and Promadhat, V.: Pulmonary Function Testing in Children: Techniques and Standards. Philadelphia, W. B. Saunders Co., 1971, 254.

A = age in years
H = height in centimeters

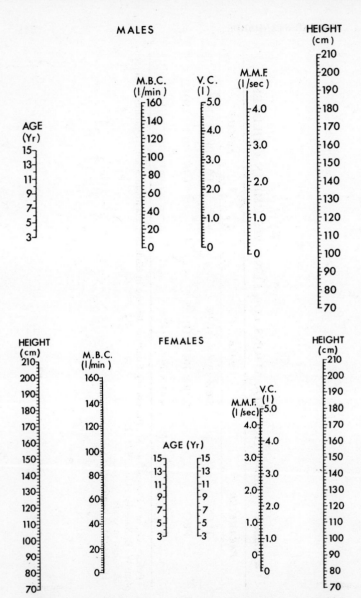

Figure 1. Nomogram for calculation of spirometry in healthy children.

Table 3 PREDICTION EQUATIONS FOR SPIROMETRY IN ADULTS

PARAMETER	MALE	FEMALE
FVC	$0.06584 \times H - 0.02954 \times A - 5.12451$	$0.05557 \times H - 0.00793 \times A - 4.89036$
$\dot{V}_{peak}$	$0.01879 \times H - 0.02406 \times A + 7.70494$	$0.05943 \times H - 0.02256 \times A - 1.23333$
$\dot{V}_{max}50$	$0.00630 \times H - 0.01831 \times A + 4.60102$	$0.02649 \times H - 0.03823 \times A - 1.72022$
$\dot{V}_{max}25$	$0.00900 \times H - 0.03540 \times A + 1.66220$	$0.00127 \times H - 0.05136 \times A + 3.60821$
$FEV_{1.0}$	$0.04525 \times H - 0.03509 \times A - 2.59946$	$0.04071 \times H - 0.02147 \times A - 2.56958$
$FEV_{1.0}/FVC$	$127.46099 - 0.24577 \times H - 0.15712 \times A$	$150.08745 - 0.36895 \times H - 0.32221 \times H$
MMF	$0.02148 \times H - 0.03384 \times A + 1.78965$	$0.02768 \times H - 0.05275 \times A + 1.38310$

Cherniack, R. M., and Manfreda, J.: Normal standards of parameters derived from the FVC maneuver in the general population. To be published.

A = age in years
H = height in centimeters

Table 4   PREDICTION EQUATIONS FOR LUNG VOLUME IN ADULTS

PARAMETER	MALE	FEMALE
VC*	$0.0481 \times H - 0.020 \times A - 2.81$	$0.0404 \times H - 0.022 \times A - 2.35$
RV*	$0.027 \times H + 0.017 \times A - 3.447$	$0.032 \times H + 0.009 \times A - 3.90$
FRC*	$0.0509 \times H - 5.1614$	$0.047 \times H - 4.853$
TLC*	$0.094 \times H - 0.015 \times A - 9.167$	$0.079 \times H - 0.008 \times A - 7.49$
FRC/TLC†	$0.18 \times A - 0.12 \times W + 52.3$	$0.16 \times A - 0.08 \times W + 45.2$

Goldman, H. I., and Becklake, M. R.: Respiratory function tests. Normal values at medium altitudes and the prediction of normal results. Amer. Rev. Tuberc., 79:457, 1959.

Grimby, G., and Soderholm, B.: Spirometric studies in normal subjects. III. Static lung volumes and maximum voluntary ventilation in adults with a note on physical fitness. Acta. Med. Scand., 173:199, 1963.

A = age in years
H = height in centimeters
W = weight in kilograms

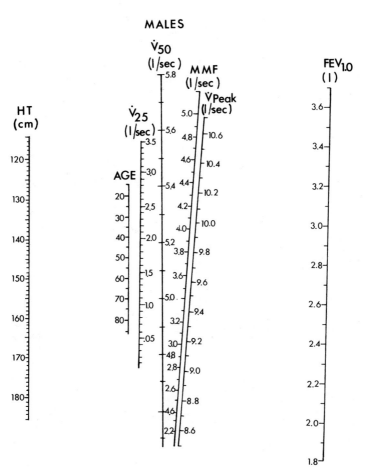

Figure 2. Nomogram for calculation of spirometry in healthy non-smoking adults.

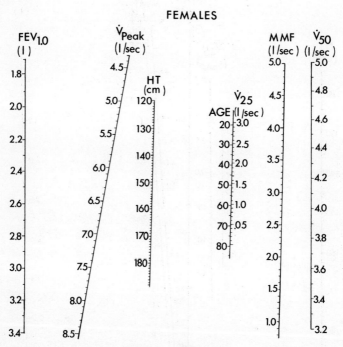

Figure 2. *Continued*

LUNG VOLUME

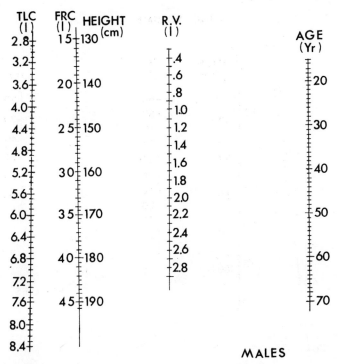

Figure 3. Nomogram for calculation of lung volume in healthy non-smoking adults.

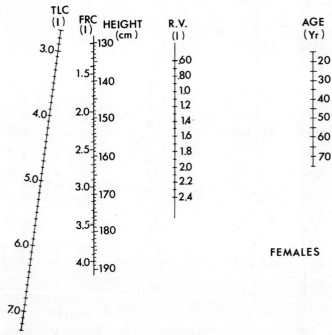

Figure 3. *Continued*

Table 5 PREDICTION EQUATIONS FOR SINGLE BREATH NITROGEN CURVE IN ADULTS

PARAMETER	MALE	FEMALE
TLC	$0.09129 \times H - 0.01281 \times A - 8.55147$	$0.07893 \times H + 0.01408 \times A - 8.21148$
RV	$0.02111 \times H + 0.01775 \times A - 2.78356$	$0.01582 \times H + 0.01368 \times A - 1.74124$
CV	$0.00871 \times H + 0.01706 \times A - 1.43627$	$0.00065 \times H + 0.1642 \times A - 0.29374$
CC	$0.02975 \times H + 0.03477 \times A - 4.20746$	$0.01639 \times H + 0.03023 \times A - 2.02821$
RV/TLC	$0.297 \times A + 11.656$	$0.190 \times A + 19.189$
CV/VC	$0.383 \times A - 0.645$	$0.454 \times A - 5.477$
CC/TLC	$0.556 \times A + 12.565$	$0.493 \times A + 16.266$
Slope III	$1.021 - 0.006 \times A$	$1.247 - 0.007 \times A$

Manfreda, J., et al.: Prevalence of respiratory abnormalities in a rural and an urban community. Submitted for publication.

A = age in years
H = height in centimeters

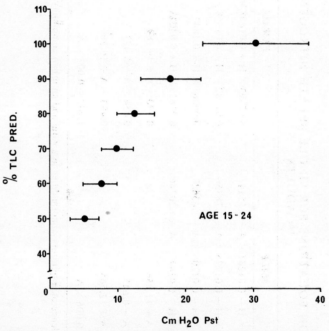

Figure 4. The expected range of the pressure-volume relationships in healthy non-smoking individuals (male and female).

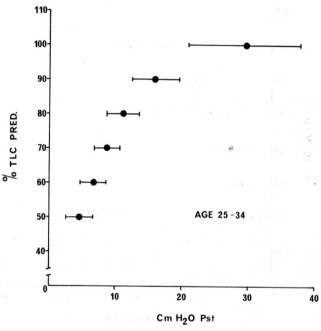

Figure 4. *Continued*

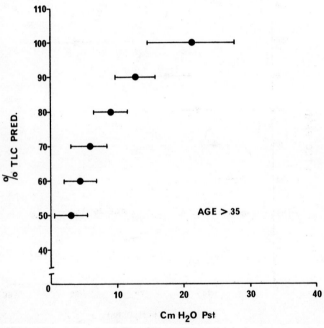

Figure 4. *Continued*

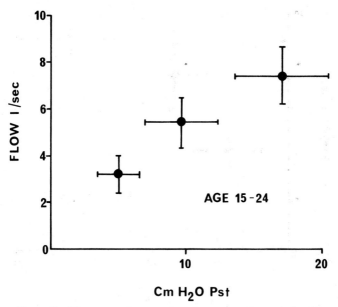

Figure 5. The expected range of static pressure-flow relationships in healthy non-smoking males.

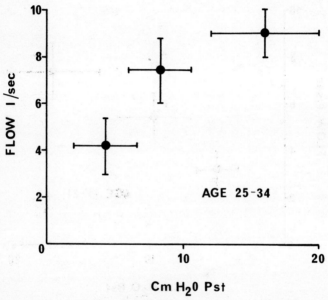

Figure 5. *Continued*

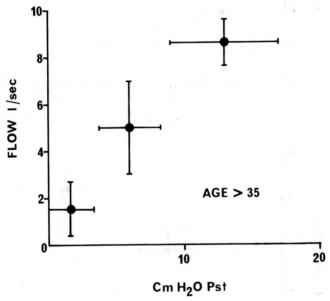

Figure 5. *Continued*

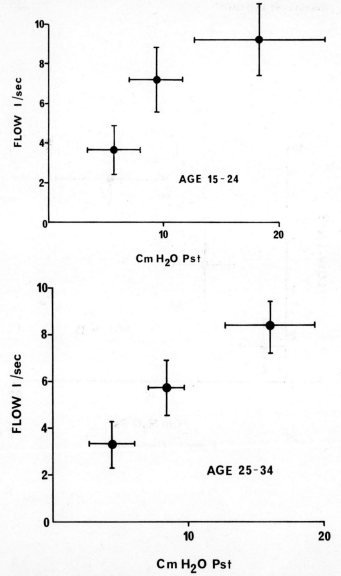

Figure 6. The expected range of static pressure-flow relationships in healthy non-smoking females.

256

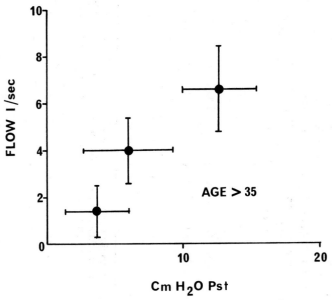

Figure 6. *Continued*

Table 6   PREDICTION EQUATIONS FOR GAS EXCHANGE IN ADULTS

PARAMETER	MALE	FEMALE
Mixing efficiency*		$-0.50 \times A + 80$
VD/VT†		$0.4 \times A + 5.1$
$D_{L_{CO}}$*	$0.0723 \times H - 0.2793 \times A + 18.167$	$0.06857 \times H - 0.252 \times A + 15.863$
% Extraction*	$82.63 - 0.13 \times H - 0.34 \times A$	$88.232 - 0.162 \times H - 0.3 \times A$
Pa_{O_2}†	$104.2 - 0.27 \times A$ (seated) $103.5 - 0.42 \times A$ (supine)	
$P(A-a)_{O_2}$†		$0.33 \times A - 3$

*Bates, D. V., et al.: Chronic bronchitis: a report on the first two stages of the coordinated study of chronic bronchitis in the Department of Veterans Affairs, Canada. Med. Serv. J. Canada, *18*:211, 1962.
†Raine, J. M., and Bishop, J. M.: A-a difference in O_2 tension and physiologic dead space in a normal man. J. Appl. Physiol., *18*:284, 1963.
A = age in years
H = height in centimeters

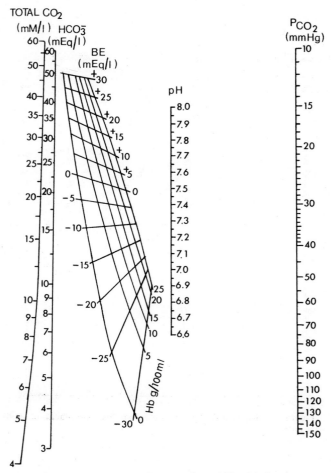

Figure 7. Nomogram for assessing acid-base balance.

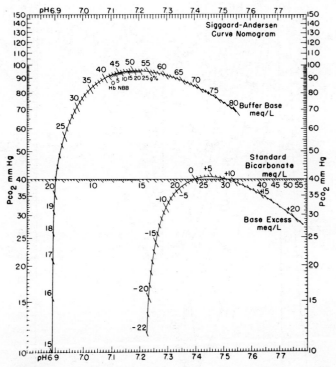

Figure 8. Siggaard-Andersen nomogram for assessment of acid-base balance.

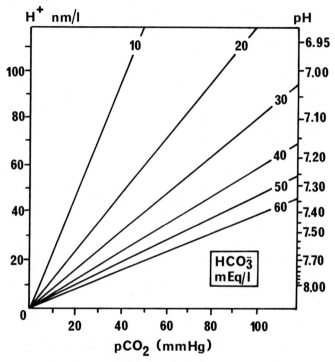

Figure 9. Nomogram for assessing acid-base balance.

SUGGESTED READING

Arbus, G. S., Hebert, L. A., Levesque, P. R., Elsen, B. E., and Schwartz, W. B.: Characterization and clinical application of the "significance band" for acute respiratory alkalosis. New Eng. J. Med., *280*:117, 1969.

Astrand, I.: Aerobic work capacity in men and women with special reference to age. Acta Physiol. Scand., Suppl. *169*: 1960.

Astrup, P., Jorgensen, K., Siggard-Andersen, O., and Engel, K.: The acid-base metabolism: a new approach. Acta Physiol. Scand., *1*: 1035, 1960.

Bates, D. V., Woolf, C. E., and Paul, G. I.: Chronic bronchitis: a report on the first two stages of the coordinated study of chronic bronchitis in the Department of Veterans Affairs, Canada. Med. Serv. J. Canada, *18*:211, 1962.

Berglund, E., Birath, G., Bjure, J., Grimby, G., Kjellmer, I., Sandqvist, L., and Solderholm, B.: Spirometric studies in normal subjects. I. Forced expirograms in subjects between 7 and 70 years of age. Acta Med. Scand., *173*:185, 1963.

Birath, G., Kjellmer, I., and Sandqvist, L.: Spirometric studies in normal subjects. II. Ventilatory capacity tests in adults. Acta Med. Scand., *173*:193, 1963.

Boren, H., Kory, R. C., and Syner, J. C.: The Veterans Administration-Army cooperative study of pulmonary function. II. The lung volume and its subdivisions in normal men. Am. J. Med., *41*:96, 1966.

Buist, A. S.: The single-breath nitrogen test. New Eng. J. Med., *293*: 438, 1975.

Buist, A. S., and Ross, B. B.: Predicted values for closing volumes using a modified single breath nitrogen test. Am. Rev. Respir. Dis., *107*:744, 1973.

Buist, A. S., and Ross, B. B.: Quantitative analysis of the alveolar plateau in the diagnosis of early airway obstruction. Am. Rev. Respir. Dis., *108*:1078, 1973.

Cherniack, R. M.: Ventilatory function in normal children. C.M.A.J., *87*:80, 1962.

Cherniack, R. M., and Raber, M. B.: Normal standards for ventilatory function using an automated wedge spirometer. Am. Rev. Respir. Dis., *106*:38, 1972.

Dickman, M. L., Schmidt, C. D., and Gardner, R. M.: Spirometric standard for normal children and adolescents (ages 5 years through 18 years). Am. Rev. Respir. Dis., *104*:680, 1971.

Goldman, H. I., and Becklake, M. R.: Respiratory function tests. Normal values at medium altitudes and the prediction of normal results. Amer. Rev. Tuberc., *79*:457, 1959.

Grimby, G., and Soderholm, B.: Spirometric studies in normal subjects. III. Static lung volumes and maximum voluntary ventilation in adults with a note on physical fitness. Acta Med. Scand., *173*:199, 1963.

Jones, N. L.: Exercise testing in pulmonary evaluation: rationale, methods and the normal respiratory response to exercise. New Eng. J. Med., *293*:541, 1975.

Jones, N. L.: Exercise testing in pulmonary evaluation. Clinical applications. New Eng. J. Med., *293*:647, 1975.

Kory, R. C., Callahan, R., Boren, H. G., and Syner, J. C.: The Veterans Administration-Army cooperative study of pulmonary function. I. Clinical spirometry in normal men. Am. J. Med., *30*:243, 1961.

Leuallen, E. C., and Fowler, W. S.: Maximum mid-expiratory flow. Am. Rev. Tuberc., *72*:783, 1955.

Lindal, A., Medina, A., and Grismer, J. T.: A re-evaluation of normal pulmonary function measurements in the adult female. Am. Rev. Respir. Dis., *95*:1061, 1967.

Macklem, P. T.: Tests of lung mechanics. New Eng. J. Med., *293*:339, 1975.

McCarthy, D. S., Spencer, R., Green, R., and Milic-Emili, J.: Measurements of closing volume as a simple and sensitive test for early detection of small airway disease. Amer. J. Med., *52*:747, 1972.

Milic-Emili, J.: Clinical methods for assessing the ventilatory response to carbon dioxide and hypoxia. New Eng. J. Med., *293*:864, 1975.

Miller, W. F., Johnson, R. L., Jr., and Wu, N.: Relationships between fast vital capacity and various timed expiratory capacities. J. Appl. Physiol., *14*:157, 1959.

Polgar, G., and Promadhat, V.: Pulmonary Function Testing in Children: Techniques and Standards. Philadelphia, W. B. Saunders Co., 1971.

Raine, J. M., and Bishop, J. M.: A-a difference in O_2 tension and physiologic dead space in normal man. J. Appl. Physiol., *18*:284, 1963.

Schmidt, C. D., Dickman, M. L., Gardner, R. M., and Brough, F. K.: Spirometric standards for healthy elderly men and women. Am. Rev. Respir. Dis., *108*:933, 1973.

Schwartz, W. B., Brackett, N. C., and Cohen, J. J.: The response of extracellular hydrogen ion concentration to graded degrees of chronic hypercapnia. The physiologic limits of the defense of pH. J. Clin. Invest., *41*:291, 1965.

Schwartz, W. G., and Relman, A. S.: A critique of the parameters used in the evaluation of acid-base disorders. New Eng. J. Med., *268*:1382, 1963.

Singer, R. B.: A new diagram for the visualization and interpretation of acid-base changes. Am. J. Med. Sci., *221*:199, 1951.

Appendix II

SELF-ASSESSMENT ANSWERS

CHAPTER 2

1. We have been given all the measurements necessary to calculate the lung compliance (C) and the flow resistance (R) at certain flow rates. In patient A the tidal volume of 800 ml was associated with a change in pleural pressure from end-expiration to end-inspiration of 2 cm H_2O. Thus the lung compliance (C) was $.800/2 = 0.400$ ℓ/cm H_2O.

   Since $C = \Delta V/\Delta P$ and ΔV was 400 ml at mid-inspiration, the pressure due to elastic resistance (P_{el}) was $\dfrac{.4 \text{ (vol)}}{.4 \text{ (C)}} =$ 1.0 cm H_2O. Thus if there were no flow resistance whatsoever, the change in pleural pressure from end-expiration to mid-inspiration would have been 1 cm H_2O. Since the pleural pressure at mid-inspiration was -7 cm H_2O, and this was a change of 5 cm H_2O from that at end-expiration, then the pressure required to overcome flow resistance (P_R) $= 5.0 - 1.0 = 4.0$ cm H_2O.

   Since the flow rate ($\dot{V}$) at mid-inspiration was 1.0 ℓ/sec, and P_R 4.0 cm H_2O, and $R = \dfrac{P_R}{\dot{V}}$, then flow resistance was 4.0/1.0 = 4 cm H_2O/ℓ/sec.

   From this data we can see that the patient has a high lung compliance (loss of elastic recoil) as well as a high flow resistance. The likely diagnosis is therefore emphysema, and we can anticipate that the patient's lungs will be overdistended with lung volume increased, and the expiratory flow rates (and $FEV_{1.0}/FVC$) reduced.

As far as patients B and C are concerned — you should now be able to deduce the correct answers for them.

2. When the lungs become fibrosed they become smaller in size (i.e., lung volume including VC is reduced) and stiffer, or more difficult to distend (i.e., compliance is low or a greater pressure is necessary to overcome elastic resistance). However, flow through the airways is not affected, so the force required to overcome non-elastic resistance will be unchanged. Since the major impedance to breathing is elastic it will be easier (i.e., less effort will be required) to breathe rapidly and shallowly. The expiratory flow rates will be low, but will be equal to or greater than those expected at any particular lung volume.

3. When the subject moves from an upright to a supine position, the diaphragm rises and the functional residual capacity falls, i.e., the resting level moves to a more expiratory position. However, the vital capacity and total lung capacity are virtually unchanged. Since the FRC has shifted to a more inspiratory position along the static pressure-volume curve, the end-expiratory pleural pressure will be less negative than it was in the upright position. As TLC and VC are unchanged, RV will be unchanged, and since FRC = RV + ERV, and TLC = FRC + IC, then ERV must diminish and IC must increase.

4. You should be able to find your own answers by referring to Figure 2–10.

5. You can also find your own answer to this question by referring to Figure 2–14.

6. Since the minute ventilation $\dot{V}_E = V_T \times f$, an increase in frequency with no change in $\dot{V}_E$ means that the tidal volume must fall, and since $V_T = V_D + V_A$ then the dead-space ventilation/min ($\dot{V}_D$) will increase. Since the tidal volume has fallen, the elastic work/breath must be less, and because the respiratory rate is more rapid and the flow rates higher, the work required to overcome flow resistance is greater. However, unless the flow becomes turbulent, the flow resistance should not be altered.

7. You shouldn't need help to answer this question by now.

CHAPTER 3

1. In the upright lung there is a pleural pressure gradient due to hydrostatic pressure, and the pleural pressure is more negative (i.e., less) at the top of the lung than at the bottom. At low lung volumes the upper region is at a different portion of its pressure-volume curve than the lower regions, and the alveoli at the top of the lung will be more distended than those near the bottom.

   Because alveolar pressure is approximately the same over all regions of lung, the amount of blood flow to any lung region is dependent on the level of the pressure of the pulmonary artery supplying that region, and this increases from the top to the bottom of the lungs. At the top or apex of the lung (zone 1), the alveolar pressure is greater than the pulmonary artery pressure and there is no blood flow. Increasing the alveolar pressure further would mean that there is a greater zone in which the alveolar pressure will be greater than the pulmonary artery pressure, and so there will be an increase in the region of lung (zone 1) in which blood flow was absent.

2. A high ventilation/perfusion ratio means that the ventilation of a region is greater than the perfusion. The gas that enters this area of lung takes little part in gas exchange, and its composition is much like that in the dead space (i.e., it is called dead-space-iike ventilation).

3. The alveolar P_{O_2} of 100 torr while the subject is breathing room air suggests that the $P_{A_{CO_2}}$ was probably normal (about 40 to 45 torr), in which case alveolar hypoventilation cannot account for the low $P_{a_{O_2}}$. In addition, since the alveolar and end-capillary P_{O_2} are virtually identical there is clearly no barrier to diffusion across the alveolocapillary membrane. Thus the difference between the alveolar (and end-capillary) P_{O_2} and arterial P_{O_2} must mean that some venous blood is being added to the blood after it left the alveoli (i.e., there is venous admixture).

4. Ligation of the artery to a lung that is still ventilated is an example of an infinite $\dot{V}/\dot{Q}$ ratio, so all the air going to that lung will be wasted and will not take part in gas exchange (i.e., the physiologic dead space increases). On the other hand, the anatomic dead space, by definition, does not change.

5. Look at Figure 3–6 again.

6. If you don't know the answer, it would probably be best if you read the chapter again.

7. $V_D = \dfrac{P_{a_{CO_2}} - P_{E_{CO_2}}}{P_{a_{CO_2}}} \times V_T$ so:

$V_D = \dfrac{40 - 20}{40} \times 600 = 300$ ml

Since the physiologic dead space is approximately 150 ml in healthy individuals, this must mean that more air is being wasted than was expected, i.e., there is ventilation of poorly perfused alveoli.

8. The diffusing capacity of gases across the alveolocapillary membrane is dependent on the surface area available for diffusion. Removal of a lung would reduce the surface area available for diffusion so the $D_{L_{CO}}$ would be less.

   Since oxygen competes with carbon monoxide for combination with hemoglobin, the $D_{L_{CO}}$ will fall whenever the oxygen concentration of the inspired gas is increased. (See Chapter 6 for the clinical applicability of this principle).

CHAPTER 4

1. The basis of this question is the Henderson-Hasselbalch equation:

$$pH = \log \dfrac{HCO_3^-}{P_{a_{CO_2}} \times 0.03}$$

a. A lower than normal $P_{a_{CO_2}}$ is indicative of a respiratory alkalosis. This may be due to primary hyperventilation, or may be a result of an increased alveolar ventilation that has been induced by a metabolic acidemia.

b. A lower than expected pH means an increase in hydrogen ion concentration (an acidemia). This can be due to a metabolic acidosis (lowered HCO_3^-) or a respiratory acidosis (high $P_{a_{CO_2}}$).

c. A high arterial CO_2 content indicates that there has been some retention of HCO_3^-. This can occur in a primary metabolic alkalosis or as compensation for an elevated $P_{a_{CO_2}}$ (respiratory acidosis).

d. A higher than normal $P_{a_{CO_2}}$ is indicative of a respiratory acidosis. This may be due to a primary alveolar hypoventilation arising from respiratory disease, or may be a result of a reduction in ventilation that has been induced by a metabolic alkalemia.

e. You should be able to answer this. It is the converse of *b*.

f. You should be able to answer this, too. It is the converse of *c*.

g. You should have been able to handle this one as well; it is the same as *c*.

2. This should be reasonably easy now. In a metabolic acidosis there is a primary reduction in bicarbonate. This alters the HCO_3^-/P_{CO_2} relationship (i.e., it is less than 20:1) so that the H^+ ion concentration rises (i.e., pH falls). The increase in hydrogen ion concentration stimulates an increase in ventilation, with a consequent rise in alveolar ventilation. This will result in a fall in $P_{a_{CO_2}}$ (provided the $\dot{V}_{CO_2}$ does not increase in a proportionate manner).

3. a. The pH is low, so there must be an acidemia present. Since the $P_{a_{CO_2}}$ is also low, it has probably been induced by an increase in ventilation, which in turn is the result of a low HCO_3^- and an increase H^+ ion concentration. In other words this is a metabolic acidemia with an associated respiratory alkalosis.

b. The pH is low normal and yet the $P_{a_{CO_2}}$ is high (i.e., a respiratory acidosis). This indicates that the primary disturbance was originally an acidosis and acidemia related to the P_{CO_2} (i.e., respiratory), and that there has been compensation by retention of bicarbonate by the kidney (i.e., a metabolic alkalosis). Thus the diagnosis is respiratory acidosis without acidemia (compensated).

c. The pH is high, so an alkalemia is present. Since the $P_{a_{CO_2}}$ is normal, the HCO_3^- must be high. Thus this is a metabolic alkalosis with alkalemia.

d. The pH is high, so an alkalemia is present. However, the $P_{a_{CO_2}}$ is inordinately high; it normally cannot rise this high in compensation for a metabolic alkalosis. Thus this is a mixed disorder, and the best bet would be that these findings indicate that the patient suffers from chronic respiratory insufficiency and has a respiratory acidosis. However, this has been complicated by the addition of a metabolic alkalosis, and the odds are that this is the result of diuretic therapy administered by the physician. Thus the diagnosis is probably respiratory acidosis with an associated metabolic alkalosis and alkalemia.

e. The pH is high, so an alkalemia is present. Since the $P_{a_{CO_2}}$ is low, it is a respiratory alkalosis with alkalemia.

4. When ketoacidosis develops as a result of diabetes, the HCO_3^- is low (metabolic acidosis), the $P_{a_{CO_2}}$ is near normal, and acidemia is present. In the examples shown in *a* and *b,* an alkalemia is present. In example *d* an acidemia is present, but this is associated with an elevated $P_{a_{CO_2}}$ (a respiratory acidosis), whereas example *e* has normal values for $P_{a_{CO_2}}$ and pH. Thus example *c,* an acidemia and a metabolic acidosis, fits the diagnosis.

5. The lungs are capable of altering the CO_2 level very rapidly through breath-holding or voluntary hyperventilation. The respiratory system does not overcompensate unless there is an added stimulus, so while the response to a metabolic

acidosis and acidemia is hyperventilation, the pH is usually only brought to around 7.35 with complete compensation. Renal retention of HCO_3^- in response to CO_2 retention is slow and takes days.

6. This is an alkalemia, and since the $P_{a_{CO_2}}$ is 48 this must be a metabolic alkalosis with an associated, though minimal, respiratory acidosis. Examples *a* and *b* would be associated with a low P_{CO_2}. Example *c* would result in a high P_{CO_2} and an acidemia, while example *e* would result in an acidemia. Clearly example *d,* in which there has been ingestion of excessive base, would produce a metabolic alkalosis and alkalemia. This in turn would inhibit ventilation, and the P_{CO_2} would rise.

CHAPTER 5

1. An ascent to a high altitude is equivalent to the inhalation of a gas mixture containing a low $F_{I_{O_2}}$. The peripheral chemoreceptors in the carotid and aortic bodies will be stimulated by the low $P_{a_{O_2}}$, so ventilation will increase and the $P_{a_{CO_2}}$ will fall. The bicarbonate will be altered very little over 10 minutes, and is therefore essentially unchanged. As a result, the HCO_3^-/P_{CO_2} ratio is altered and the pH will rise. Since we haven't heard that the hemoglobin content is altered in any way, its capacity to carry oxygen is unchanged.

2. a. CO_2 inhalation results in a rise in P_{CO_2} and an increase in ventilation. The elevated P_{CO_2} will induce a fall in pH, while the P_{O_2} will rise because 25 per cent O_2 is being inhaled.

   b. Acute respiratory acidosis develops when the alveolar ventilation falls. By definition this is an elevated CO_2 tension that is associated with a fall in P_{O_2} (unless a high oxygen concentration is being inhaled), and since it is acute, the pH will be lower than normal.

    c. The low $F_{I_{O_2}}$ means that the $P_{a_{O_2}}$ will be low. This will stimulate ventilation and therefore lower the P_{CO_2} and raise the pH.

    d. Since the metabolic acidosis is no longer associated with an acidemia, there has been compensation by hyperventilation and a lowering of $P_{a_{CO_2}}$. There is a minimal rise in $P_{a_{O_2}}$. Since we have been told there is no acidemia, the pH is within normal range.

    e. Voluntary hyperventilation implies an increase in alveolar ventilation, which results in a fall in $P_{a_{CO_2}}$ and a rise in pH. The $P_{a_{O_2}}$ rises minimally.

    f. Alveolocapillary block implies a diffusion difficulty for oxygen. This results in a fall in $P_{a_{O_2}}$. The low $P_{a_{O_2}}$ stimulates ventilation, so the P_{CO_2} falls and pH rises.

3. Initially on a subject's reaching an altitude, the low $P_{a_{O_2}}$ stimulates an increase in ventilation with a consequent fall in P_{CO_2} and an alkalemia. After a while compensation occurs through increased renal excretion of HCO_3^-, so that the HCO_3^- is low. By the time the subject returns to sea level, the pH is probably high normal. On return to sea level where $F_{I_{O_2}}$ is higher, the $P_{a_{O_2}}$ rises and ventilation is no longer stimulated by hypoxemia, so it falls and the $P_{a_{CO_2}}$ rises to normal levels. However, since the HCO_3^- was low, this would result in a picture resembling a metabolic acidosis with acidemia.

4. The carotid and aortic bodies are stimulated by a drop in $P_{a_{O_2}}$. The $P_{a_{O_2}}$ is not altered by *a*, *b*, or *c*, but will fall at altitude.

5. A noticeable increase in ventilation occurs when the $F_{I_{O_2}}$ falls to less than 0.14. The increase in ventilation results in a fall in $P_{a_{CO_2}}$. The P_{CO_2} in the cerebral tissues also falls because CO_2 is freely diffusible across the blood-brain barrier. On the other hand, the blood-brain barrier is relatively impermeable to HCO_3^-, so the HCO_3^- in the brain remains unaltered. As a result a tissue alkalemia develops.

CHAPTER 8

Patient Examples

1. a. The static pressure-volume curve of the lungs is shifted downward and to the right, i.e., the slope is reduced, which means that the lung compliance is diminished.

   b. The absolute flow rates are low, but in fact they are higher than expected at this low lung volume because the driving pressure of the lung is increased (i.e., compliance is low).

   c. Since the lung volume is reduced, this is indicative of a restrictive defect. Of course, this is confirmed by the measurement of lung elastic recoil.

   d. Example *1* is a metabolic acidosis, and there is no reason to suspect that this is present. Example *3* is alveolar hypoventilation with respiratory acidosis and acidemia. This is not found commonly in a patient suffering from a restrictive disorder. Example *2*, i.e., hypoxemia with a low $P_{a_{CO_2}}$ (respiratory alkalosis) and alkalemia, is a fairly common finding in patients suffering from restrictive disorders.

   e.-g. you decide.

2. Let's look at Patient A first:

   a. The $P_{I_{O_2}}$ was $20.94 \times (747 - 47) = \simeq 147$ torr.
      Then the $P_{A_{O_2}} = 147 - (36 \times 1.25) = 102$ torr, and the $P(A\text{-}a)_{O_2} = 102 - 52 = 50$ torr.

      The V_D/V_T ratio $= \dfrac{36 - (.04 \times 747 - 47)}{36} = \dfrac{36 - 28}{36} = \dfrac{2}{9}$

   b. Since the $P_{a_{CO_2}}$ is normal, there is no alteration in alveolar ventilation and thus no respiratory acidosis or respiratory alkalosis. The diffusing capacity is normal, as is the dead space $(2/9 \times 480) = <110$ ml. When the $F_{I_{O_2}} = 1.0$, the $P_{a_{O_2}}$ was 550 torr, so there is no true shunt. Clearly mismatching of ventilation and perfusion in the lung is present, and the hypoxemia must be due to perfusion of poorly ventilated alveoli.

Patients B and C should present no problems, and the reader should be able to deduce the answers for them.

3. a. In this patient the lung volumes are markedly reduced, so a restricture disorder is present. The flow rates are also low, but are they lower than one would expect at these particular lung volumes (i.e., is there also an obstructive disorder)? If you draw out the flow-volume envelopes and compare the flow rates at the appropriate lung volume, you will be able to determine whether this is a mixed disorder.

   b. Since the $P_{a_{CO_2}}$ is not elevated there is no alveolar hypoventilation; in fact, alveolar hyperventilation must be present. The $P_{A_{O_2}}$ breathing air is $147 - (30 \times 1.25) \simeq 109$, and the $P(A\text{-}a)_{O_2}$ therefore is $109 - 40 = 69$ torr. This is a markedly increased $P(A\text{-}a)_{O_2}$. It does not appear to be due to a diffusion defect ($D_{L_{CO}}$ was 90 per cent of predicted) or a true shunt, because the $P_{a_{O_2}}$ rose to 520 torr on 100 per cent O_2. Thus the hypoxemia was most likely due to a mismatching of ventilation and perfusion in the lungs.

   c. After oxygen therapy was instituted, the $P_{a_{O_2}}$ rose. However, assessment of the $P_{a_{O_2}}$ without consideration of the $F_{I_{O_2}}$ and the $P(A\text{-}a)_{O_2}$ may be misleading, and does not tell you whether there has been improvement. As you can see, the $F_{I_{O_2}}$ was .24 before the sample at 1 hour, and .28 before the next arterial blood sample at 2 hours. However, it was maintained constant between the second and third hours.

   Let us look at what happened to the A-a gradient during this time. When higher oxygen concentrations than room air are being inhaled it is not really necessary to correct for RQ when calculating the $P_{A_{O_2}}$, but let's do it anyway, because omitting this correction would not alter the conclusions.

At 1 hour, the $P_{A_{O_2}}$ was $.24 \times (747 - 47) = 168 -$ about $48 = 120$ torr.
Thus the $P(A\text{-}a)_{O_2}$ was $120 - 60 = 60$ torr.

At 2 hours, the $P_{A_{O_2}}$ was $.28 \times (747 - 47) = 196 - 50 = 146$ torr.

Thus the $P(A\text{-}a)_{O_2}$ was $146 - 70 = 76$ torr.

At 3 hours, the $P_{A_{O_2}}$ was $196 - 30 = 166$ torr, and the $P(A\text{-}a)_{O_2}$ was $166 - 80 = 86$ torr. Thus we can see that even though the $P_{a_{O_2}}$ was higher between hours 2 and 3, there was actually a deterioration of gas exchange.

   d. After 3 hours the pH was higher than normal, and this is not surprising because a respiratory alkalosis exists.

4.   a. This little girl has hypoxemia and respiratory acidosis (i.e., $P_{a_{CO_2}}$ is elevated) as well as an acidemia.

   b. The $P_{a_{O_2}}$ is about $147 - (75 \times 1.25) = 52$. Thus, the A-a gradient is $52 - 35 = 17$ torr. This is somewhat greater than might be expected if alveolar hypoventilation alone were present.

   c. Thus, in addition to alveolar hypoventilation a coexistent disorder, possibly a ventilation/perfusion imbalance, is probably present as well.

   d. When 100 per cent oxygen was inhaled, the $P_{a_{O_2}}$ was > 500 torr, indicating that no true venous admixture was present.

   e. After 36 hours of treatment, the $P_{a_{CO_2}}$ was 44 torr at a time when alkalemia was present. Since the $P_{a_{CO_2}}$ is within the normal range, the alkalemia must be due to a metabolic disorder.

You should be able to answer the next two parts by now.

5.   The findings are of an increase in lung volumes, so the patient's lungs are hyperinflated. Despite the high lung volumes, the maximal expiratory flow rates are lower than expected, so it is likely that the flow resistance is increased.

However, remember that the flow resistance $(R) = \dfrac{P}{\dot{V}}$,

and so $\dot{V}$ may be low if the driving pressure is low (i.e., if the patient has lost lung elastic recoil), even if flow resistance is normal.

Hyperinflation of the lungs is frequently associated with an increase in flow resistance, and this may occur in patients suffering from emphysema, bronchitis, or asthma.

After the administration of a bronchodilator, the patient has less air trapping (RV is lower) and is breathing at a lower lung volume (FRC). This is important when considering the effect of a nebulized bronchodilator. The expiratory flow rates that are reported are essentially the same, but since the vital capacity is now bigger and the RV smaller, the flow rates must be compared at equivalent lung volumes in order to determine whether there is an objective improvement following the bronchodilator. Thus flow-volume envelopes have to be compared. If you did this and found that the flow rate at a particular volume was increased, then one could infer that flow resistance improved following the bronchodilator, and that their use is clearly indicated.

6. a. On admission to hospital, the patient's pH was 7.26. Thus an acidemia was present. Since the P_{CO_2} was high, this was a respiratory acidosis with acidemia.

   b. By definition, an elevated $P_{a_{CO_2}}$ is indicative of alveolar hypoventilation. To determine whether there is an associated disturbance one must calculate the $P(A-a)_{O_2}$. The $P_{A_{O_2}}$ is about 77 torr and the $P(A-a)_{O_2}$ about 42 torr. Since pure alveolar hypoventilation does not lead to an increase in $P(A-a)_{O_2}$, there must also be some $\dot{V}/\dot{Q}$ imbalance.

   c. The post-cardiac arrest analysis of the arterial blood indicates that the acidemia is still present. However, the $P_{a_{CO_2}}$ is now within normal limits, so a metabolic acidosis and acidemia must be present.

   d. Since the $P_{a_{CO_2}}$ is normal, we know that there is no alveolar hypoventilation. However, marked $\dot{V}/\dot{Q}$ mismatching must be present because the $P(A-a)_{O_2}$ is about 51 torr.

   e. Even though the $P_{a_{O_2}}$ has risen from 35 to 40 torr, we have seen that the $P(A-a)_{O_2}$ rose from 42 torr to 51 torr.

f. On the third day, arterial blood analysis indicated that the metabolic acidosis and acidemia persist.

g. Since the $P_{a_{CO_2}}$ is still normal, no alveolar hypoventilation exists. However, the $P(A-a)_{O_2}$ is now about 60 torr, so there is probably even greater mismatching of ventilation and perfusion.

h. The $P_{a_{O_2}}$ is higher, but so is the $F_{I_{O_2}}$. The increase in A-a gradient suggests that gas exchange may be deteriorating.

i. On day 6 the arterial blood data indicate that the patient is now alkalemic and, since the $P_{a_{CO_2}}$ is normal, one can deduce that a metabolic alkalosis and alkalemia must be present.

j. Once again the $P_{a_{CO_2}}$ is normal, and the $P(A-a)_{O_2}$ is now about 58 torr.

k. The $P_{a_{O_2}}$ is higher, but the A-a gradient has changed little.

7. This is the last case example. By this time you don't need me. Why don't you answer these questions all by yourself?

INDEX

Page numbers in *italic* type refer to
illustrations; (t) denotes tables.

277